AF687867

HEADACHES

Why You Have Them
What You Can Do About Them

Egilius L. H. Spierings, MD, PhD

Copyright © 2026 Egilius L. H. Spierings, MD, PhD
All rights reserved
First Edition

Fulton Books
Meadville, PA

Published by Fulton Books 2026

Cover Design: Sven E. J. Spierings, MS, MBA

ISBN 979-8-90270-027-2 (paperback)
ISBN 979-8-88731-922-3 (hardcover)
ISBN 979-8-88731-921-6 (digital)

Printed in the United States of America

To the memory of Harold George Wolff (1898–1962) and John Ruskin Graham (1909–1990), in whose footsteps I followed, and to my lovely granddaughters, Cayleigh Naomi Spierings and Leah Isabella Spierings, who I hope one day will follow in my footsteps

My other neighbor, who is sitting on my left in the bus, is different because he does not say much and seems distant. He draws everybody's attention, because people here are usually very open and talkative, happy to tell stories or express opinions about everything. The only thing he has told me until now is that he does not work and that he has difficulty working. What sort of difficulty? He is not saying.

Eventually, however, when the forest grows smaller and finally disappears behind us, which means that we are approaching Kumasi, he decides to confess something to me. He has a problem. He is sick. He is not sick all the time, only sometimes, periodically. He has been to a number of local specialists, but none of them is able to help him. The matter is that in his head, under his skull, there are animals.

It is not that he sees them, thinks about them, or is afraid of them, not at all. Nothing of that sort. The problem is that they are in his head, they live there; they run around, graze, hunt, or just sleep there. When they are gentle kind of animals, like antelopes, zebras, or giraffes, he can bear their presence very well; they are even pleasant. However, sometimes a hungry lion appears. He is hungry and furious, so he roars. The roar of this lion splits his skull.

—*Ebony* by Ryszard Kapuściński

Contents

Preface

A play called *The Cherry Orchard* written by the Russian physician Anton Chekhov and first performed in 1904 contains the following aphorism or truism: "If there is an illness for which people offer many remedies, you may be sure that particular illness is incurable." In relation to headache, we could rewrite this as follows: If there is a medical complaint for which people offer many remedies, you may be sure that particular complaint is unmanageable.

I am convinced that people who have turned to medicine for the treatment of their headaches can attest to the accuracy of this statement. Physicians or other health care practitioners throw treatments at them, seemingly willy-nilly, sometimes several at once and, unfortunately, often with deplorable results.

Headaches are part of life, and when intense, the problem is generally that of migraine, a genetically determined and inherited vulnerability. As such, headache, including migraine, we cannot cure, and management is all that we can offer. When I trained in the diagnosis and treatment of headache (and face pain), it was appropriately called headache management.

Now we generally refer to this medical specialization as headache medicine, an inherent promise that we as physicians or other health care practitioners generally cannot fulfill. After all, the word *medicine* comes from the Latin word *medicina*, the verb root of which is *mederi*, meaning "to heal."

What turns headache into a medical complaint is generally its intensity. The intensity of headache is much more a driver of medical consultation than is frequency, and migraine is by far the most common reason for us to have intense headaches.

Not only do people offer many remedies for migraine, there is also an abundance of theories regarding this medical condition.

Here, another literary statement comes to mind, which the English physician Richard Gordon wrote in his book *The Alarming History of Medicine*, published in 1983: "The history of medicine is largely the substitution of ignorance by fallacies." Of course, this is an exaggeration, but there is definitely some truth to it when it comes to migraine, which some have called the happy hunting ground for theoreticians.

Over time, we have advanced many different theories regarding the nature of migraine and published them in high-end medical journals. In most cases, the people who developed them, often physicians, had very little experience, if any, dealing with migraine from a clinical perspective. Sometimes, they advanced them for the single purpose of self-aggrandizing, increasing the importance of their research, or promoting the sales of a product.

What I describe in *Headaches* has its basis in extensive study and training as well as in decades of work in medical practice, academic and private, dedicated to the diagnosis and treatment of headache and face pain. In addition, it is based on the management of thousands of patients, many of whom I followed for years, if not decades.

Introduction

Migraine

Headaches are such a common experience that anybody who claims never to have had one we can rightfully assume has poor memory. Approximately half of the population has headaches at least once per month, approximately 15 percent at least once per week, and approximately 5 percent daily. However, how much people suffer from the headaches they experience, of course, also depends on their intensity.

Fortunately for most people, headaches are of an intensity that nonprescription pain medications, like aspirin, acetaminophen, also called paracetamol, ibuprofen, or naproxen, fully relieve them. Approximately half of the general population with daily headaches is that fortunate; the other half has daily headaches with migraine headaches superimposed upon them.

Migraine headaches are intense headaches that the nonprescription pain medications mentioned do not relieve, at least not fully, although they certainly can provide some benefit. Those who have migraine headaches need medications that have the power to relieve them *fully*. These are usually not just pain relievers but medications specifically developed for the treatment of migraine.

Tension and Sinus Headache

Migraine is by far the most common reason for people to experience headaches that are not relieved by a couple of aspirin. Headaches of this intensity occur in approximately 20 percent of the population, which means that one out of five people has at least one such intense headache in the course of a year.

Some may say that their intense headaches are tension headaches, and others may consider them sinus headaches. However, bad tension headaches, bad sinus headaches, and bad hangover headaches do not exist. They are all migraine headaches caused by tension or stress, nose or sinus issues, or alcohol.

Migraine is a genetically determined and inherited condition that makes people vulnerable to intense headaches. As it is genetic, it runs in families; therefore, one only needs to inquire with parents, grandparents, or siblings about headaches that are not relieved by a couple of aspirin. Men especially tend to hide behind bad tension headaches or bad sinus headaches, whereas, in fact, they have migraine.

Brain Disease

Of course, there are also other causes of headache than migraine, including causes of intense headaches. What people are generally concerned about, however, is that their headaches are due to something ominous going on in the brain. This is a valid concern, but it is, fortunately, rare to have headaches due to brain disease, especially considering how very common they are.

What we often forget is that headaches can also be due to disorders unrelated to the brain, affecting the body as a whole, such as high blood pressure, or hypertension; shortage of red blood cells, or anemia; and low thyroid function, or hypothyroidism. These conditions can also aggravate migraine, and when they cause intense headaches, it is due to the presence of the aforementioned genetically determined and inherited migraine vulnerability.

Certainly, diseases of the brain can cause intense headaches, but that is rare without a migraine vulnerability. In addition, we have wonderful imaging techniques available to examine the brain and make sure that it is in good shape. Therefore, when you have headaches, intense or not, there should be no reason to worry. The imaging techniques are readily available, and your physician or other health care practitioner can easily order them for you, covered by your insurance.

This Book

If you have headaches, intense or not, you will want to know why you have them, and what you can do about them. This is what this book is all about, and I wrote it for you, the one with the headaches. Headache is a complicated problem, to which I have dedicated my entire professional life, spanning almost half a century.

I trained in headache management with John R. Graham, MD, MACP, who also spent his entire professional life, more than half a century, studying and treating headaches. Professor Graham, in turn, trained with someone whom I would like to call the father of headache research, Harold G. Wolff, MD.

In the first half of the last century, Professor Wolff extensively investigated headache in most of its presentations and causes. In fact, much of what we know today about headache, migraine or otherwise, we know from his research conducted in headache patients.

In this book, I will elaborate on the various presentations and causes of headache. I will delve into the treatment as well, very much based on my training with Professor Graham.

Medical management involves the diagnosis and treatment of the patient and their complaints. The diagnosis involves more than ordering tests, and the treatment constitutes more than writing out one or more prescriptions. Both require caring for the patient, which means providing reassurance about the nature of the complaints and educating them as to the cause or causes and about the various aspects of the treatment.

Please note that the book contains a glossary of medical terms behind the Acknowledgments section.

Chapter 1

Do I Have a Brain Tumor?

Tumor

In all likelihood, you do not, but it is an important question to ask and one that medicine should take seriously and address adequately, because reassurance is key. In the question, brain tumor does not just stand for a tumor in the brain, which can be cancer but does not have to be.

Tumor in medicine is a general term for swelling, which can be due to a number of causes and, again, does not have to be cancer. In the brain, any swelling of significance causes headache, because a hard structure, the skull, surrounds it and does not give. Within the skull, swelling increases the pressure, and that is painful, although generally not terribly.

The swelling can be in part of the brain or between the brain and the skull, but it can also affect the brain as a whole. When the latter is the case, we call it benign intracranial hypertension or, better, idiopathic intracranial hypertension. We also refer to it as pseudotumor cerebri, because it presents as a brain tumor while it is not.

We see idiopathic intracranial hypertension, or IIH, most commonly in obese young women, and the cause is generally unknown. A blood clot in one of the big veins draining blood from the brain can be the reason for the swelling. Occasionally, the cause is the use of tetracycline, an antibiotic, or taking too much vitamin A, an old-fashioned treatment for acne. It typically causes persistent, low-grade headache, associated with impaired vision due to swelling of the optic discs.

The optic disc is the site of entry of the optic nerve in the back of the eye. We can inspect it by examining the eye ground, which is part of a physical examination called fundoscopy, important in the context of evaluating a patient with headache.

The optic nerve is an extension of the brain and swells when the pressure in the skull is increased. Thus, looking into the eyes and examining the eye grounds is an important way of obtaining reassurance that a brain tumor, or anything else that increases the pressure in the skull, is not the cause of the headaches.

Apart from general swelling of the brain or a brain tumor, increased pressure can be due to enlargement of the chambers of the brain, called hydrocephalus. Other causes of increased pressure in the skull are the presence of blood in or around the brain or a brain abscess.

Imaging

A much better way of addressing the brain tumor question than by examining the eye grounds through fundoscopy is to visualize the brain through techniques, such as computerized tomography (CT) or magnetic resonance imaging (MRI).

When we use computerized tomography to picture the brain, no contrast is required if the headache is acute and bleeding is what we want to exclude. Bleeding can result from injury to the head, from a stroke, also called brain attack, or from rupture of an aneurysm of a brain artery, which is a localized expansion that looks like a little balloon.

The rupture of such a little arterial balloon is a catastrophic event and is associated with headache that comes on like a blow to the head. In medicine, we call a headache that comes on this way—that is, like a blow to the head—a headache of very acute or peracute onset or a thunderclap headache. It is characteristic of a condition called subarachnoid hemorrhage, which is a bleeding between the two inner membranes surrounding the brain. It presents a medical emergency, because half of the people who suffer from it unfortunately die.

If we perform computerized tomography of the brain for reasons other than to exclude bleeding, as in the case of post-traumatic headache or headache of peracute onset, we should do it with intravenous iodine contrast. This is important in case a suspected blood vessel abnormality, such as an arteriovenous malformation, or AVM, causes the headaches.

An arteriovenous malformation is a congenital abnormality that is present at birth. When affecting the brain, it can manifest itself as migraine—in this case, migraine with aura. It is usually present in the back of the brain, where vision is located, and the resulting aura symptoms are visual in nature.

Aura symptoms in the context of migraine originate in the brain and occur before the onset of the headache or during the initial phase of headache development. They are either visual in nature, affecting vision on one side or the other; somatosensory, affecting sensation on one side of the body or the other; or involve speech.

In case of an arteriovenous malformation in the back of the brain, a so-called occipital arteriovenous malformation, the aura symptoms are visual in nature, and the resulting disorder is that of symptomatic migraine with visual aura. The following patient vignette is an example of an occipital arteriovenous malformation manifesting as migraine.

A thirty-seven-year-old man has been experiencing headaches since college. Five years ago, they occurred once per month; after that, two or three times per year. However, over the last ten days, he experienced them five times.

The headaches come on during the day, usually in the afternoon, build to their maximum intensity in five to ten minutes, and last six to twelve hours. They are located on the left, in the forehead and behind the eye. The headaches feel like an intense pressure, and in half of them, the pain is severe. They are associated with light sensitivity and, occasionally, also with nausea and vomiting.

A visual disturbance precedes the headaches by ten to twenty minutes, consisting of blue spots in the right visual field. The visual disturbance lasts for the duration of the headaches. Bright light, overexertion, red wine, monosodium glutamate (MSG), and drinking more than two cups of coffee bring on the headaches.

Brain magnetic resonance imaging revealed a large arteriovenous malformation in the left occipital lobe. With a special procedure, surgeons made it smaller, causing permanent loss of vision in the process. Unfortunately, the headaches continued unabated, along with the visual disturbance.

Superior to computerized tomography of the brain is magnetic resonance imaging. When performed to address the brain tumor question, it does not require intravenous contrast, in this case gadolinium. As opposed to brain computerized tomography, it does not involve radiation, which is an advantage as well. Finally, it has better resolution, as we call it, allowing more detailed examination of the brain, including its blood vessels, the nerves originating from the brain stem, and the membranes surrounding it.

The brain itself is insensitive to pain, and therefore, any condition affecting it must be big enough to stretch its blood vessels, which are pain sensitive, to cause headache. Generalized swelling of the brain will do this, as well as enlargement of the chambers of the brain, or hydrocephalus. A tumor in the brain, whether cancer, bleeding, or abscess, will do it too, also as a result of associated swelling due to edema. Inflammation, usually from a viral infection, so-called viral encephalitis, also causes headache through localized or generalized swelling of the brain.

Meninges

In contrast to the brain, the membranes surrounding it, the meninges, three in total, are sensitive to pain like the brain blood vessels. The two inner membranes can become inflamed because of a viral, bacterial, or fungal infection called meningitis. This is a concern particularly in young children, teenagers, and adolescents.

In this case, the headache is associated with fever and with a particular kind of stiffness of the neck. This particular neck stiffness makes it difficult to bend the neck forward while it moves well in every other direction. We encounter the same kind of neck stiffness with subarachnoid hemorrhage, which is a bleeding between the two inner membranes of the brain. However, in the latter, there is no fever, and the headache has a very acute or peracute onset, like a blow to the head.

Bleeding can also happen between the two outer membranes surrounding the brain and between the outer membrane, called dura mater, and the skull. When it occurs between the dura mater and the skull, a so-called epidural hematoma, it is always due to a head injury, generally one that is impactful enough to fracture the skull. This is not the case when the bleeding happens between the two outer membranes of the brain, called a subdural hematoma. In this case, a head injury still causes the bleeding, but it is generally mild and, hence, easily forgotten.

Subdural hematoma predominantly occurs in the elderly, in whom shrinkage of the brain stretches the veins between the brain and the skull. This makes these so-called bridging veins vulnerable to injury, and a mild head injury, such as knocking the head against an open cabinet door, can cause them to bleed. The result is a venous bleed, which by its very nature is not as catastrophic as the arterial bleed from an aneurysm in subarachnoid hemorrhage. It generally causes a persistent, low-grade headache, which may be accompanied by memory impairment.

If we do not consider the possibility of a subdural hematoma in an older patient with recent-onset headache, we will fail to diagnose it. It may then be fatal, although we can easily detect it with the aforementioned imaging techniques and treat it with a relatively simple surgical procedure.

The outer membrane of the brain, the dura mater, can also be the source of a tumor, which is generally a benign tumor called meningioma. It is slow growing, develops over years or decades, and can manifest itself as chronic headache, including migraine. If it presents as migraine, it would be migraine without aura, and the condition would be that of symptomatic migraine without aura. The following patient vignette is an example of a meningioma manifesting as chronic tension headache.

A thirty-three-year-old woman has been experiencing headaches for seven years, initially occurring infrequently and mild in intensity. Over time, they gradually increased in frequency and have been almost daily for the last year. The almost daily headaches usually come on around noontime and are worst in the late afternoon or early evening. They are generally located in the right forehead but sometimes across the forehead. The headaches are not associated with nausea, vomiting, light sensitivity, or noise sensitivity.

Computerized tomography of the brain with iodine contrast revealed a meningioma in the front of the head, located on the right. Removal of the tumor resulted in resolution of the headaches.

Children

In children, brain tumors are often located in the small brain, or cerebellum, which is the part of the brain that resides in the back of the head and plays an important role in equilibrium. These tumors grow over weeks or months, ultimately compressing the fourth brain chamber, through which the brain fluid emerges from the chamber system.

The medical term for brain fluid is cerebrospinal fluid, or CSF, which is made in the chambers of the brain called lateral ventricles. The cerebrospinal fluid passes through the brain stem to the fourth brain chamber, or fourth ventricle, on its way flowing through the third ventricle, which is in the brain stem as well but in the front while the fourth ventricle is in the back.

The fluid emerges from the ventricular system in the brain and brain stem via the roof of the fourth ventricle and is absorbed in the blood through the veins on top of the brain. When something compresses the fourth ventricle, for example a tumor, the brain fluid cannot emerge from the ventricular system, and the chambers, or ventricles, enlarge to cause what we call hydrocephalus.

Hydrocephalus renders severe headaches, often associated with so-called projectile vomiting. They typically happen at night, waking the child from sleep or causing them to wake up in the morning with severe headache. Although the occurrence of headaches at night is something that we encounter in adults with nocturnal migraine or cluster headache, it is an ominous presentation in a child, requiring expeditious action in terms of brain visualization, preferably consisting of magnetic resonance imaging.

Sometimes, viral meningitis is mistaken for migraine, but here we are dealing with a single episode while migraine comes in repeated episodes, also referred to as attacks, over a longer period. With bacterial meningitis, such a mistake is unlikely to happen, because the patient is very sick with high fever and may be confused or even delirious. In both circumstances, a physician should perform a spinal tap or lumbar puncture for proper diagnosis, but not before picturing the brain with computerized tomography or magnetic resonance imaging.

Elderly

In an older patient with a relatively recent onset of headaches, subdural hematoma is not the only concern; we also need to consider two other medical conditions, namely, temporal arteritis and ophthalmic zoster.

Temporal arteritis, better termed giant cell arteritis, is a disorder that causes inflammation of the body's arteries including those of the head, leading to persistent, generally low-grade headache, often associated with fatigue, low-grade fever, and muscle pain. The muscle pain may happen particularly in the jaw muscles while chewing, which we refer to as jaw claudication.

We diagnose the condition through blood tests of inflammation, measuring the erythrocyte sedimentation rate, or ESR, and the C-reactive protein, or CRP, level. We confirm the diagnosis by microscopically examining a section of the blood vessel that runs in the temple—the superficial temporal artery.

Although the headache may be on one side only, it is prudent to take sections of both temporal arteries. These sections need to be relatively long, because the inflammation may not affect the entire length of the arteries.

Blindness and stroke are potential consequences of giant cell arteritis. Treatment requires the long-term intake of a corticosteroid and, hence, the need for solid confirmation of the diagnosis. We follow progress in treatment by repeating the aforementioned blood tests of inflammation.

Ophthalmic zoster is a presentation of shingles, which is due to reactivation of the chicken pox virus residing in the body. The virus inhabits nerve knots, known as ganglia—in this case, the so-called sensory ganglia, of which the trigeminal ganglion is one.

The trigeminal ganglion is located in the skull, at the base of the brain, and has three branches, hence the name trigeminal (tri = three). These are the ophthalmic branch, the maxillary branch, and the mandibular branch, which carry sensory information from the forehead, cheek, and jaw respectively to the brain.

We have a trigeminal ganglion on either side, each with a trigeminal nerve, and with ophthalmic zoster, the ophthalmic branch of one of them is inflamed. This causes pain on one side or the other of the forehead because of reactivation of the chicken pox virus in the trigeminal ganglion. Little blisters develop in the painful area, singularly or in small groups, several days after the onset of the pain. Sometimes, the blisters are difficult to see because they are hiding among the eyelashes or in the hairline.

The treatment of ophthalmic zoster is with an antiviral medication, like acyclovir or valacyclovir, and with a medication for nerve pain, such as gabapentin or pregabalin. It is also important to follow up with an eye specialist, or ophthalmologist, because the condition may affect the cornea and, therefore, can cause blindness.

Chapter 2

If Not from Brain Tumor, Why Do I Get Headaches?

Stress

Almost everyone experiences headaches; as mentioned, approximately half of the population gets them at least once per month, approximately 15 percent at least once per week, and approximately 5 percent daily.

We often attribute headaches to stress, but that is only a small part of the story; many things cause them, and the list is long. Stress is certainly at the top of the list, along with not eating on time, fatigue, and lack of sleep. Weather changes in the sense of impending rain or snow are high on the list as well, related to changes in barometric pressure.

The system in the body that is sensitive to barometric changes is the sinus system. It consists of two sinuses in the cheeks, the maxillary sinuses; two in the forehead, the frontal sinuses; several small ones in the nose, the ethmoid sinuses; and a large sinus in the base of the skull, the sphenoid sinus.

The sinuses communicate with the outside world via the nose through small openings, which are often narrow and, hence, easily blocked. When these communications are not perfectly open, the sinuses cannot readily adapt to changes in barometric pressure, which causes stress in the sinus system and, consequently, headache.

The stress that I am referring to here is physical stress. It is, of course, not the mental one that people generally associate with the word *stress*. Headache may be the body's response to stress in general, whether it is mental or physical.

However, I do not believe that stress, whatever its nature, is the biological trigger of headache which, in my opinion, is fatigue. I think that headache's biological function lies in its relation to fatigue, functioning as a secondary symptom. In other words, when we ignore fatigue, headache is the complaint that emerges, further forcing us to take a step back.

Fatigue

We often look at fatigue as a mental symptom, and when it is continuous or persistent, we consider it an indication of depression. I personally believe that this is wrong and that fatigue is very much a physical symptom, indicating a lack of metabolic energy.

Metabolic energy is the energy that our body makes from nutrients and that our cells need to function. Without the necessary energy, they cannot do whatever they are supposed to do; when it comes to important cells related to headache, the nerve cells and muscle cells, they cannot relax.

Energy metabolism is a cyclical activity in the sense that we build energy as we sleep and use it during the day, when we are awake and functioning. Building energy is the function of sleep, and related to it, it is important not only how long we sleep but also when we sleep.

For our body to produce enough energy, we need to sleep at the right time; everyone with jet lag experience knows this. You can sleep as long as you want, but if it is not at the right time in your sleep-wake cycle, you will continue to feel tired. Under those circumstances, you experience a lack of metabolic energy, and your body will direct whatever energy is available to the vital organs.

The vital organs include the brain and the heart, for sure the most essential ones, and also the lungs, liver, spleen, and kidneys. Not on the list are the muscles, other than the heart muscle, which comprise more than a third of our body weight but are not directly relevant for survival. With lack of metabolic energy, muscle cells literally cannot relax, because they cannot restore the electrical charge across their outer membranes, which allows them to relax.

The muscles that suffer the most when metabolic energy is in short supply are those that have the highest energy requirement. These are the so-called postural muscles that keep our body erect. They include those in the back of the neck that keep our head up, the muscles in the lower back that keep our pelvis up, and the calf muscles that keep our legs perpendicular to our feet. The jaw muscles, interestingly, are part of this muscle system as well; they counteract gravity when the body is erect, preventing our mouth from dropping open.

Tension Headache

When it comes to headache in relation to fatigue, I think that the muscles in the back of the neck play a crucial role. These are the so-called posterior neck muscles or posterior cervical muscles. Tightness of those muscles is invariably associated with that of adjacent muscles, which are the muscles in the head, jaws, shoulders, and upper back. Muscle tightness causes tenderness, soreness, or pain; the muscles may feel thickened, hard, or beset with taught bands.

When the muscles in the head tighten, the soreness or pain causes headache, typically involving the head as a whole and of mild or mild to moderate intensity. This is what people generally call headache, regular headache, stress headache, or tension headache. A physician or other health care practitioner may refer to it as muscle contraction headache or tension-type headache.

The International Headache Society (IHS) introduced the term "tension-type headache" in its classification for two reasons. First, studies of muscle activity in general do not demonstrate contraction of head muscles when this kind of headache is present. However, this may be due to studying the wrong muscles, using the wrong study technique, or employing a technique that is not sensitive enough to register muscle activity. Second, agreement exists that tension, or mental stress, is not the only cause of this type of headache but that it can be due to a great variety of causes.

The causes of tension headache are tremendously mundane, making it such a common experience that we may easily consider it part of life. Fortunately, such headaches typically do not last more than a couple of hours and are easily relieved by rest or relaxation or by taking a nonprescription pain medication. If these treatments generally do not provide relief, they are almost certainly not regular headaches, or tension headaches, and migraine is the most likely problem.

An exception exists when those headaches are present daily or almost daily, lasting most of or all day. Then we refer to the disorder as chronic muscle contraction headache, chronic tension headache, or chronic tension-type headache, which accounts for the headaches in approximately half of those afflicted with daily headaches.

I mentioned earlier that approximately 5 percent of the population has headaches daily. In half of them, it concerns this particular condition—that is, chronic tension headache—and nonprescription pain medications provide modest, if any, benefit, and it is merely temporary.

Chronic Tension Headache

Chronic muscle contraction, tension, or tension-type headache, whatever you call it, is a disorder characterized by low-grade headache that is present most of or all the time. We used to consider it a depression equivalent, which means depression presenting with continuous, low-grade headache rather than as feeling down in the dumps.

I do not know what this assumption is based upon, and it may be nothing more than the idea that when you have headaches most of or all the time, you must be depressed. This specific consideration is what led to the study of amitriptyline in the treatment of what I like to call chronic tension headache.

Amitriptyline is a so-called tricyclic, the first of its kind, introduced in the early 1960s for the treatment of depression. Relatively shortly afterward, we showed it to be beneficial in the treatment of chronic tension headache. We still use it for this purpose, taken once daily at bedtime—once daily because it works long and at bedtime because it causes sedation.

The latter improves sleep if there is a problem sleeping through the night; otherwise, it likely causes daytime drowsiness or fatigue. For this reason, I prefer not to prescribe it when sleeping is not an issue. If falling asleep is also a problem, the patient can take it two hours before bedtime to help that as well.

The dose of amitriptyline is much lower for headache prevention than it is for the treatment of depression. We no longer prescribe it for depression, because we have more effective, better-tolerated, and safer medications available. A good starting dose is ten or twenty-five milligrams at bedtime, if needed, increased slowly with intervals of a month or longer to allow ample time for proper assessment of its benefit.

For the treatment of headache, I like to increase the dose until there is some dryness of the mouth, but I do not want the mouth to be cotton dry. This indicates that enough medication is in the body to have a so-called anticholinergic action, which is associated with muscle relaxation. In order to see the dry mouth, we generally do not need to increase the dose beyond fifty to one hundred milligrams per day. By comparison, for the treatment of depression, we used to prescribe it in daily dosages of two hundred to four hundred milligrams.

The aforementioned sedation is due to a so-called antihistaminic effect, and amitriptyline has a proserotoninergic action as well. The latter means that it makes more of the neurotransmitter serotonin available in the brain. Initially, we thought this to mediate its antidepressant effect, but we now believe that it is the reason it relieves pain, including headache. Therefore, it may work in two ways to improve chronic tension headache—one being an anticholinergic muscle relaxant action and the other a proserotoninergic effect, relieving pain.

Apart from drowsiness and dry mouth, amitriptyline can cause constipation, which is a potential side effect, similar to dry mouth, of its anticholinergic action. However, more significant than any of those side effects is weight gain, because it is not resolved upon discontinuation of the medication. This is the reason I avoid prescribing it to women, especially, of course, if there is already a weight problem.

The weight gain with amitriptyline comes with increased appetite and sweet craving and is due to facilitation of insulin release from the pancreas. This is the hormone set free by the ingestion of carbohydrates that acts by clearing glucose from the blood and putting it into storage.

In diabetes mellitus, this hormone is lacking partially or fully, which results in blood glucose levels so high that it ends up excreted in the urine. This is also the basis of the term *diabetes mellitus* with *diabetes* referring to copious urination and *mellitus* to the sugar in the urine. One of the symptoms of undiagnosed and untreated diabetes mellitus is unexplained weight loss, the opposite of what we see with a medication like amitriptyline—"unexplained weight gain."

If the patient with chronic tension headache does not have a problem falling asleep, sleeping through the night, or waking up early, I prefer not to prescribe amitriptyline. As mentioned, I also avoid it in women or in anyone actually who is even slightly overweight. Under those circumstances, I prescribe a related tricyclic called imipramine, for which there is evidence of benefit in chronic tension headache as well.

However, imipramine is not as effective as amitriptyline, but patients tolerate it better with fewer side effects. I still recommend that they take it once daily at bedtime, and the dosing is the same as for amitriptyline. In addition and if necessary, I gradually increase the dose until there is some dryness of the mouth. It causes less sedation than amitriptyline and, consequently, less daytime drowsiness or fatigue.

Fatigue is an important side effect when treating headaches, because it can cause them, as explained earlier. It is paramount to monitor in headache patients with any medication, because it may increase headache frequency. Fatigue is a common side effect of medications in general even if they do not specifically cause sedation. It is a nonspecific side effect, because they are toxic to the body and do not belong there.

Imipramine causes less constipation than amitriptyline and less weight gain, although both may still be an issue.

Hypothyroidism

A common medical condition that can cause chronic tension headache is low thyroid function, or hypothyroidism. It affects approximately 5 percent of the population and occurs more often in women than in men. It runs in families as Hashimoto's thyroiditis, which is a so-called autoimmune disorder in which the body makes antibodies against the thyroid gland. These antibodies cause inflammation of the thyroid gland, which in turn makes it underactive or overactive, but more often the former than the latter.

Continuous, also called persistent, low-grade headache is a symptom of low thyroid function in approximately a third of patients. However, in medicine, we rarely recognize it as such. In general, we often do not recognize hypothyroidism either, mainly because its complaints are rather nonspecific.

Since thyroid function regulates energy metabolism, fatigue is the most direct result of low thyroid function due to decreased energy metabolism. However, fatigue has numerous causes. In combination with the fact that it is common, patients and physicians or other health care practitioners alike often ignore it.

Patients frequently attribute it to stress, and physicians and other health care practitioners often ascribe it to depression. However, as far as I am concerned, neither is true. In fact, I think that the most common cause of fatigue is actually lack of restorative sleep.

As explained, energy metabolism is a cyclical activity: we build energy as we sleep and spend it while awake. Producing energy is the function of sleep, and related to it, as aforementioned, it is important not only how long we sleep but also when we sleep. Hence, for us to produce enough energy, we need to sleep sufficiently long and at the right time.

In order to build enough energy to last the day, I recommend at least eight or nine hours of sleep per night, which also needs to be uninterrupted to be restorative. Thyroid function determines the rate of energy metabolism, which is the rate at which sleep builds energy. The lower the thyroid function, the more sleep we need, which should be at the right time and uninterrupted to produce sufficient energy to last the day.

If we do not have enough energy, we feel tired; along with it, we feel cold, we crave sweets, and our muscles are tight. We feel cold because our body tries to save energy by preserving heat. I compare it to turning off the heaters in the bedrooms during the winter, which for the body means decreasing circulation in the nose, hands, and feet.

We crave sweets because carbohydrates provide a quick and energetically cheap way of making metabolic energy. For the body, however, fat is actually the best source of energy, because on a weight basis, it provides the most. Our muscles are tight when we lack metabolic energy and feel tired, because in contrast to what people generally think, muscles need energy to relax, not to contract.

Apart from fatigue and continuous, or persistent, low-grade headache, cold intolerance and dry skin are symptoms of hypothyroidism as frequently as headache is. In addition, scalp hair becomes brittle, and loss of eyebrow hair, especially at the sides, is a characteristic sign as well.

Thyroid Function

We can easily determine thyroid function by measuring the levels of two hormones in the blood, which are the thyroid-stimulating hormone, or TSH, and levothyroxine, or T4. The former comes from the pituitary gland at the base of the brain, and as the name implies, it stimulates the thyroid gland to make and release its hormones.

The thyroid gland synthesizes two hormones—triiodothyronine, or T3, and the aforementioned levothyroxine, or T4. The latter is, in fact, a so-called prohormone, which is converted—mostly in the liver but also in other cells of the body—into the active thyroid hormone triiodothyronine.

In contrast to triiodothyronine, levothyroxine is a hormone that lasts long in the blood, making its level relatively stable. Therefore, instead of measuring triiodothyronine, which is short lasting, we prefer to determine the levothyroxine level to assess thyroid function.

In the past, we just measured the level of thyroid-stimulating hormone because it was easier to determine and interpret than those of triiodothyronine and levothyroxine. That is why, generally, we still evaluate thyroid function by measuring the thyroid-stimulating hormone level only. However, I think that this does not provide the full picture, and that we should determine the levothyroxine level as well.

We should measure its free level, referred to as free T4, or FT4, as opposed to the total level, or TT4. In addition, when thyroid disease runs in the family, which can be underactive or overactive thyroid, we should measure the level of thyroid peroxidase antibody, or TPO-a, as well. The latter is elevated in Hashimoto's thyroiditis, which is a potential diagnosis that we would otherwise miss.

Reference Range

Any blood test performed in a laboratory comes with a so-called reference range, often erroneously called normal range. We do not know the latter for any blood test done in a laboratory, simply because we are not born with a manual in our hands. The reference range of a given test is always specific to the laboratory that performs the test, based on a large number of samples tested—for example, obtained from a blood bank.

The laboratory subsequently assumes that the test results have a so-called normal distribution and calculates the mean or average, along with the standard deviation. It then subtracts two times the standard deviation from the mean to obtain the low number of the reference range and adds two times to it to determine the high number.

Accordingly, the laboratory provides the results of any test it performs with a reference range that includes 95 percent of the results obtained from a large number of samples tested. Does this sound like anything that comes even close to deserving the name "normal range?" It is a construct by a particular laboratory exclusively for use in relation to a specific test it performs.

Another issue of at least equal importance is the aforementioned assumption of a normal distribution. This means that you find approximately as many results below the mean or average as above it. That may be true for some tests, but it certainly does not apply to all, and definitely not for the tests to determine thyroid function. The reason for this is simply that low thyroid function is much more common than high thyroid function, at least by a factor five.

With the above elaborate explanation, I aim to make clear that interpreting the results of a thyroid function test—or any test, for that matter—is not as easy as people often assume. It certainly involves more than just considering the results in relation to the reference ranges.

Focusing on evaluating thyroid function, I wrote tests, not just the thyroid-stimulating hormone level but the free levothyroxine level, or FT4, as well and, if indicated, also the thyroid peroxidase antibody, or TPO-a, level.

Inverse Relation

Thyroid-stimulating hormone is a pituitary hormone, and levothyroxine is a thyroid hormone. It is important to know that these two glands, the pituitary gland and the thyroid gland, interact with each other in a negative feedback relation. This means that when the thyroid-stimulating hormone level increases to stimulate thyroid function, the released levothyroxine decreases it in response. As a result, the levels of those two hormones should be such that if one is relatively low, the other is relatively high and vice versa.

We determine whether a level is relatively high or relatively low depending on where it is in relation to, or relative to, the reference range. Consider the thyroid-stimulating hormone level relatively high and the free levothyroxine level relatively low, thus existing in an inverse relation to each other. How high should the thyroid-stimulating hormone level be or how low should the free levothyroxine level be to diagnose underactive thyroid, or hypothyroidism?

Amazingly enough, we do not know, but some suggest that a thyroid-stimulating hormone level above 3.5 micro-international units per milliliter should be considered an indication of hypothyroidism. Considering the numbers in the context of the patient's complaints, which is what we really should be doing for correct interpretation of laboratory results, is not that easy with hypothyroidism, because the symptoms are so nonspecific.

The situation is even more daunting to interpret when the levels of both hormones—thyroid-stimulating hormone and levothyroxine—are relatively low, in and by itself an abnormal situation. Especially here, a trial treatment with levothyroxine, the thyroid hormone that we prescribe to treat hypothyroidism, can provide valuable insight. Adding it to the body should decrease the thyroid-stimulating hormone level, and if this happens, the situation as it exists is probably normal for the patient.

However, I have often seen that, under those circumstances and in response to a test dose of levothyroxine, the thyroid-stimulating hormone level goes up, which is also definitely abnormal. Increasing the dose will ultimately bring it down, creating a situation in which the thyroid-stimulating hormone level is relatively low and the levothyroxine level relatively high.

This is what I aim for in my treatment of hypothyroidism—bringing the thyroid-stimulating hormone level down to around 0.5 micro-international units per milliliter while keeping the levothyroxine level within the reference range.

Menstruation

A symptom I often find helpful in the context of evaluating the results of thyroid function testing is menstrual abnormalities. Based on what I have seen in treating women with levothyroxine for hypothyroidism, the menstrual cycle/menstruation complex is quite sensitive to thyroid hormone deficiency.

An abnormality of the menstrual cycle exists when menstruation does not happen regularly on a monthly basis. It can occur too frequently, for example every two weeks, which we call polymenorrhea, or not frequently enough, for example every two to three months or even less called oligomenorrhea.

Abnormalities of menstruation include periods that are long or heavy, called menorrhagia or hypermenorrhea, or that are painful, called dysmenorrhea. For general information, when a long or heavy (vaginal) bleeding occurs unrelated to menstruation, for example in menopause, we call it metrorrhagia.

When menstrual cycle or menstruation abnormalities are present, the likelihood of abnormal thyroid function is increased. The thyroid function can be low or high, with underactive thyroid, or hypothyroidism, much more common than overactive thyroid, or hyperthyroidism. With treatment of hypothyroidism, even with a small amount of levothyroxine prescribed, such as twenty-five or fifty micrograms per day, correction of the menstrual cycle or menstruation abnormality is often the first improvement seen.

An elevated level of thyroid peroxidase antibody, or TPO-a, suggests Hashimoto's thyroiditis, which is an autoimmune disease that runs in families. It can manifest itself as hypothyroidism or hyperthyroidism but, again, more often as the former than the latter. The levels of thyroid-stimulating hormone and levothyroxine in the blood may be within the reference ranges. Nevertheless, I am a proponent of treating it as hypothyroidism with levothyroxine. In approximately half of the patients in whom I have proceeded this way, I observed the level of the antibody to come down, sometimes dramatically.

I do not know whether this is important or not, but at one time people considered the antibody toxic to the brain and the cause of a disorder known as Hashimoto's encephalopathy, with *encephalopathy* being a broad term for brain disease.

Hemoglobin

Thyroid function regulates energy metabolism, and when it is low, fatigue ensues. Energy metabolism, of course, needs substrates—that is, fuel; however, it also requires oxygen, vitamins, and minerals.

Hemoglobin, which is the material in the red blood cells that colors them red, acquires the oxygen needed for energy metabolism in the lungs and carries it around the body. Low hemoglobin, a condition referred to as anemia, is a common cause of fatigue. It lowers energy metabolism by depriving it of oxygen, which it needs to burn the substrates, the fuel, to make energy.

When measuring hemoglobin, the same issue arises as discussed earlier in relation to the reference range. Again, the latter is laboratory specific, and we cannot and should not equate it with normal range. In contrast to thyroid function, I have an optimal level for hemoglobin that I like to see in patients, which is approximately 13.5 grams per deciliter for women (8.4 millimoles per liter) and approximately 15 grams per deciliter for men (9.3 millimoles per liter). If it is lower than that, I will investigate it further as to the cause and treat it, if possible.

In order to manufacture hemoglobin, the body needs vitamins and minerals, particularly vitamin B_{12}, also known as cobalamin, and folate or folic acid, sometimes referred to as vitamin B_9, as well as iron. Vitamin levels are easily determined in the blood, and we best assess iron availability in the body through the ferritin level.

Ferritin is a protein in the blood that contains iron and, as such, provides information about the body's iron reserve. I like its level to be at least sixty to eighty nanograms per milliliter, based on the recommendation by the World Health Organization (WHO) for women of childbearing potential.

The vitamin B_{12} level I prefer to see above three hundred picograms per milliliter, and the folate or folic acid level above twenty nanograms per milliliter. When these vitamin levels are low, I suggest one thousand micrograms of vitamin B_{12} per day and one milligram of folate or folic acid, both available without prescription.

When the ferritin level is not where I like it to be, I generally treat that with a nonprescription medication containing forty-five milligrams of iron in the form of ferrous sulfate. Depending on the level, I recommend one or two tablets per day, preferably taken with food. Most patients tolerate this dose well without side effects, like nausea or constipation. If the latter is an issue, I combine it with a nonprescription stool softener, called docusate, in a dose of one hundred or two hundred milligrams per day.

I treat the ferritin level independent of the hemoglobin level even if the latter is where I like it to be, which has demonstrated benefit in improving energy and treating fatigue. Iron is an important mineral in energy metabolism and in the manufacturing of hemoglobin alike.

Much more often than due to a lack of vitamin B_{12} or folate or folic acid, low hemoglobin is due to a shortage of iron, referred to as iron-deficiency anemia. Hence, low levels of hemoglobin and ferritin often occur together, and an iron supplement treats both. However, before initiating treatment, it is paramount to determine the cause of the low hemoglobin or low ferritin. If the reason is other than diet, adding iron to the body is not going to solve the problem, and we may even be missing a serious medical condition. An important and often overlooked explanation of a low hemoglobin level, low ferritin level, or both is loss of blood from the stomach.

Stomach

When the stomach bleeds acutely, it is most often from an ulcer either in the stomach or in an adjacent part of the esophagus. It is evident that this is the problem, because we vomit blood or observe the stool turning tarry black.

The stomach can also bleed chronically, however, and this is something that we would not necessarily be cognizant of. It is quite common, especially in people who have headaches frequently, due to the use of nonprescription or prescription pain medications.

Pain medications come in three categories: acetaminophen or paracetamol; aspirin and related medications called NSAIDs; and opioids, sometimes still referred to by the old term: narcotics. The acronym NSAID stands for nonsteroidal anti-inflammatory drug, and its plural is NSAIDs. These are medications to treat inflammation, not related to cortisone. The latter is a naturally occurring corticosteroid, or steroid for short, that we have employed for the treatment of inflammation since the 1950s.

Corticosteroids are very potent anti-inflammatory medications, and well-known examples are dexamethasone and prednisone. In contrast to the nonsteroidal anti-inflammatory drugs or NSAIDs, they do not treat pain because they lack analgesic properties. Nonsteroidal anti-inflammatory drugs, in contrast, treat inflammation *and* pain and do so very effectively but, potentially and with regular use, at the cost of irritating the stomach.

Such irritation leads to a condition referred to as chronic gastritis, characterized by tiny ulcerations that we call micro-ulcerations, which can progress to stomach ulcers. These micro-ulcerations bleed and cause minimal blood loss in the stool that we cannot see. Over time, however, it leads to a lowering of hemoglobin and ferritin levels and, thus, to iron-deficiency anemia.

The occult blood loss, as we call it, that we cannot see, we can easily detect with a simple stool test. Any physician or other health care practitioner can perform it in the office; it is simple and cheap.

Gastritis

Chronic gastritis can be silent or asymptomatic, which means without complaints. This is especially the case when caused by the chronic use of nonsteroidal anti-inflammatory drugs, or NSAIDs. When it does cause symptoms, I find that medicine often does not fully appreciate them for their significance and potential impact on the patient's health.

Acid complaints are common, ranging from heartburn, a burning sensation in the pit of the stomach, to reflux, in which the burning extends behind the breastbone to the throat. These symptoms are worse after a particularly sour drink, such as orange juice, grapefruit juice, or tomato juice, or after tomato-rich, often Italian, or greasy food.

In addition, they are generally worse at night, when the body is in a horizontal position, making reflux easier to occur. With or without heartburn or reflux, there can be pain in the stomach area, which is the area of the abdomen immediately below the breastbone. In medicine, we refer to this part of the belly as epigastric area.

Least recognized as manifestations of chronic gastritis are chronic nausea and so-called restaurant syndrome. As the name implies, the former refers to the daily or almost daily occurrence of nausea. When accompanied by daily or almost daily headaches, patients often erroneously attribute the nausea to the headaches. However, a rule of thumb is that when daily or almost daily nausea accompanies daily or almost daily headaches, the nausea is not from the headaches but from a stomach problem.

Restaurant syndrome is different from Chinese restaurant syndrome, which is caused by the eating of food that contains monosodium glutamate, or MSG. The symptoms of Chinese restaurant syndrome include, among others, headache, light-headedness, nasal congestion, facial pressure, and jaw tightness.

In contrast, eating any big or heavy meal brings about restaurant syndrome, resulting in a pressing urge to move the bowels. People with this particular problem do not like to eat in restaurants because of the bowel movement urgency that follows on the heels of finishing a meal. It is due to an exaggerated gastrocolic reflex, caused by the irritation of the stomach, the gastritis.

The gastrocolic reflex connects the stomach (*gaster* in Greek) with the large bowel (*colon* in Latin), and its activation causes the large bowel to move, resulting in a bowel movement. Stomach irritation exaggerates this reflex, as is the case in chronic gastritis, but the same is true when the large bowel is irritated, as in irritable bowel syndrome, or IBS. Especially with the latter, the urgent bowel movement is associated with acute-onset abdominal bloating and cramps.

Irritable bowel syndrome, by the way, is a chronic condition of constipation, diarrhea, or both, in which the bowel movements are preceded by abdominal bloating and discomfort or pain. These belly symptoms typically resolve after the occurrence of the bowel movement or movements.

We diagnose chronic gastritis based on the complaints and on examination of the abdomen and of the stool, the latter for occult blood, as explained, and based on the findings, we determine the seriousness of the condition. Additional testing is usually not required, but if despite treatment the symptoms persist or the stool continues to be positive for occult blood, a gastroenterologist should perform endoscopic examination of the stomach for ulcers.

Proton-Pump Inhibitors

We treat chronic gastritis with a so-called proton-pump inhibitor, or PPI, of which several are available, including esomeprazole, lansoprazole, omeprazole, pantoprazole, and rabeprazole. These are prescription medications, but some of them are also obtainable without prescription, such as lansoprazole and omeprazole.

It is important that we use the proton-pump inhibitor in a high enough dose and that we continue the treatment for a sufficient length of time to ensure healing of the lining of the stomach. The dose should be high enough to eliminate the complaint, whether it is heartburn, reflux, stomach pain, or chronic nausea.

With a satisfactory high dose, these symptoms should resolve within days or, at most, in a week or so, but their relief does not mean resolution of the problem. For the lining of the stomach to heal fully, the patient needs to discontinue the offending pain medication or medications and take the proton-pump inhibitor for at least six to twelve months. It is also important that on treatment, the stool is and remains negative for occult blood.

Proton-pump inhibitors heal the lining of the stomach by powerfully suppressing acid secretion. They generally do not have side effects, and patients can take them long-term without ill effects, although some people claim differently.

The nonsteroidal anti-inflammatory drugs, or NSAIDs, weaken the lining of the stomach so that the acid irritates it more easily. The caffeine present in many pain medications, especially those for the treatment of headache or migraine, contributes to their negative impact. Caffeine is a relatively long-acting medication that constricts the blood vessels in the head to relieve headache, but it also stimulates acid secretion in the stomach.

If the use of a proton-pump inhibitor, or PPI, is associated with the development or worsening of constipation, this is not a side effect but an indication that the stomach is healing and that its impact on the large bowel, through the gastrocolic reflex, has diminished.

If there is constipation or a history thereof, I often initiate constipation treatment along with prescribing the proton-pump inhibitor. I do so with the stool softener docusate in a dose of one hundred or two hundred milligrams per day. If necessary, I add senna at bedtime, two tablets of 8.6 milligrams each.

Alternatively, I may use magnesium citrate in the form of 200-milligram tablets, starting with one tablet per day and going up to four, if indicated. It is important that the patient takes the constipation treatment, whatever it is, daily and that the dose allows for daily or almost daily bowel movements with stool of as normal consistency as possible.

Muscles

As explained earlier, fatigue causes headaches by not allowing the head muscles to relax due to a lack of metabolic energy. Stress makes them contract, and the general wear and tear of the day does the same. Thus, even without stress making the head muscles tight, fatigue causes headache. For example, this is the case in hypothyroidism, which can manifest itself with a continuous, or persistent, low-grade headache.

We generally do not realize either that something as simple and common as reading or watching television is a muscular effort that can make the head muscles tight. These activities in particular tighten the forehead and neck muscles, sometimes leading to the vertical creases in the center of the forehead, known as glabellar lines.

Glabella refers to the ordinarily smooth area of skin between the eyebrows, just above the bridge of the nose. It contains the procerus and corrugator muscles, which are so-called accessory muscles of accommodation. They support the muscles of accommodation, which are the small muscles in the eyeballs that surround the lenses, called ciliary muscles.

In order for us to focus on anything closer than twenty feet, or six meters, the ciliary muscles need to contract to make the lenses rounder. We ordinarily read at a distance of one or two feet, which is approximately thirty to forty-five centimeters. Consequently, quite a bit of contraction is required; if they have a hard time managing, the procerus and corrugator muscles contract to assist them. The problem is worse when reading on a computer monitor or watching television, because focusing in a fixed vertical plane is additionally strenuous to the eyes.

Reading on a computer monitor strains the muscles in the back of the neck as well, the so-called posterior neck muscles or posterior cervical muscles. Apart from involvement in head posture, in particular keeping the head straight on the neck, and neck movement, these muscles also strongly connect to the eyes. Just try to move your eyes without moving your head or neck, and you will see how difficult that is due to the strong functional connection between them.

Sleep

I already explained that we build energy as we sleep at night and spend it as we are awake and functioning during the day. Therefore, it is easy to understand why lack of sleep is a cause of headache, simply because it causes fatigue. In order for the body to have enough energy to last the day, we generally need eight or nine hours of uninterrupted sleep, occurring at the right time.

Unfortunately, oversleeping in the morning can also cause headache, very much a feature of migraine, which is more a relaxation-type headache than a stress-type headache. This means that when caused by stress, it is more likely to develop after the stress, when relaxation follows, than during it.

With regard to sleep, the consequence of the above is that for a migraineur to get enough sleep, eight or nine hours per night, oversleeping in the morning is not an option. It requires retiring in a timely fashion, preferably at approximately the same time each night, and the same applies to rising in the morning. Regularity is key when migraine is your vulnerability—unfortunately not only with sleep but with pretty much anything else as well.

Not eating on time, along with stress, fatigue, and lack of sleep among the most common causes of headache, is less easy to explain. It may have to do with the associated relatively low blood glucose level with this particular sugar being a source of fast energy. In this context, it is interesting to note that diabetes mellitus, a medical condition in which blood glucose levels are consistently high, seems protective of headache.

Menstrual Cycle

An important cause of headaches in women not mentioned yet is the menstrual cycle. Despite the fact that it is paramount in the context of migraine, its underlying mechanism is not known. It is so significant that I would say that if we understood why women experience headaches in relation to the menstrual cycle, we would have a handle on at least half of humanity's headache suffering.

In relation to the menstrual cycle, headaches are particularly likely to happen premenstrually—that is, in the days leading up to menstruation—midcycle at the time of ovulation, and at the tail end of menstruation. At these times, when women are most vulnerable to headaches, the blood estrogen level changes. It goes down premenstrually and at the time of ovulation, and it starts to rise again at the tail end of menstruation.

Estrogen is not one hormone but several, the most important ones being estradiol, estriol, and estrone. They are essential to the sexual and reproductive health of women. Regarding the menstrual cycle, they are important in ovulation and menstruation while the other female hormone, progesterone, is of particular significance in menstruation.

Chapter 3

With Intense Headaches, Do I Have Migraine?

Headache Intensity

You probably do, no matter how you define intense, and there are several ways of defining it. You could just consider the intensity of the headaches, which we assess on a three-point scale or on a ten-point scale.

The three-point scale rates headache intensity as mild, moderate, or severe. We relate these intensities to the extent in which the headaches affect the ability to function physically, realizing that even minimal pain affects mental functioning. If the headaches do not impact physical functioning, we refer to them as mild. If they affect the ability to function physically but do not require bed rest, we consider them moderate. If they require bed rest, we refer to them as severe.

Trying to get an idea of headache intensity, I generally ask patients, "How often do you have headaches, and how often are they intense?" In order to add some objectivity, I will follow up by asking them how often headaches happen that require lying down, even if only shortly.

The ten-point scale allows applying a number to the headache intensity, with ten being the worst pain possible. I employ that scale when I am trying to get information on the headaches, a little more detailed in terms of their intensity—for example, at the time of treatment or after treatment.

We can also define headaches as intense based on their response, or lack thereof, to treatment with nonprescription pain medications.

A third way is to consider the association of the headaches with symptoms, such as nausea or vomiting. Only headaches of moderate to severe or severe intensity are generally accompanied by nausea, and only severe headaches cause vomiting.

After an assessment of the overall headache burden, I ask patients how often the headaches are associated with nausea and how often with vomiting. More specifically, I will ask, "Out of ten headaches, how many come with nausea and how many with vomiting?"

A final way of assessing headache intensity is by asking how often they wake the patient from sleep at night, knowing that only severe headaches do so.

Of course, headaches fluctuate in intensity, and not all headaches that a given person experiences are necessarily the same. Migraine headaches do occur in all intensities, and can even be mild, but the problem generally arises when they are moderate or severe.

Under those circumstances, they are disabling and require bed rest, also because of nausea or vomiting. The accompanying stomach complaints add to the suffering as well as to the disability, the latter because they are sensitive to movement and require lying down as motionless as possible.

Nonprescription pain medications may relieve migraine headaches to the extent that the pain is bearable, the stomach feels better, and physical functioning is feasible. However, they rarely, if ever, relieve them fully and to the point that the head is clear again, which is the goal of acute or abortive migraine treatment. We can generally achieve this goal only with prescription medications specifically developed for the treatment of migraine.

Tension and Sinus Headache

Of course, migraineurs not only have the intense headaches of migraine but also, like everyone else, get tension headaches. In addition, they may experience another common type of headache, sinus headache which like tension headache, is of mild intensity.

Sinus headache is really a misnomer, because it involves face pain rather than headache, located centrally in the face. Frequently, it is not even pain but more a discomfort or pressure, which patients have described to me as the feeling of a plunger placed in the center of the face. It is similar to their describing tension headaches as the sensation of a band pulled tight around the head.

The problem with migraineurs is that, whatever headache they get, it easily develops into a migraine headache. This is where a lot of confusion exists, and terms like *tension migraine* and *sinus migraine* found their origin. Both are nonsensical terms that we better avoid because, if anything, they add to the confusion of which there is already plenty around when it comes to migraine.

Just to reiterate, tension headaches, also called stress headaches, muscle contraction headaches, or tension-type headaches, are headaches of mild intensity that feel like a band tightened around the head. Sinus headaches—or more correctly, sinus face pain—are a similar pressure feeling but involving the nose and cheeks, the center of the face, as if a plunger sits on it. Anything beyond those tension or pressure sensations means development into migraine in terms of headache, which is important because of what it implies for treatment.

We prefer that people not treat tension or sinus headaches with pain medications, or analgesics, although generally, that is what they do. It is better to treat tension headaches with rest, relaxation, and heat applied to the neck and shoulder muscles, acknowledging cause and mechanism. Sinus headaches, we should treat with an intranasal antihistamine or intranasal corticosteroid to shrink the lining of the nose and open up the communications from the nose to the sinuses.

Once a tension or sinus headache develops beyond a tightness or pressure sensation and becomes a real headache, we should treat it with an abortive migraine medication for best benefit. The same is true for hangover headaches, which of course we avoid best by not drinking at all or, at least, not drinking excessively. Like tension and sinus headaches, they are mild headaches; bad hangover headaches are migraine headaches brought on by alcohol, and we should treat them as such.

Migraine

When you have intense headaches, it is very reasonable to assume that you have migraine, and you should seek medical care accordingly. Migraine is by far the most common cause of such headaches, especially if you have been getting them for some time. It is a chronic condition, which is genetically determined and inherited. In my opinion, it is not a disease but a vulnerability to intense headache, however defined.

Migraineurs get headaches from the same causes as everyone else. The difference is the intensity and, thus, the impact on personal, social, and professional life, as well as on health, mental and physical, which is why treatment is *always* required.

The focus of the treatment is with medications and, hence, pharmacological, which is most effective with those specifically developed for migraine. Although they are generally safe for long-term use and well-tolerated, they require prescriptions in most countries and, thus, medical consultation.

Nonprescription medications with a migraine label are not specific to migraine and have the same ingredients as their nonmigraine counterparts. As far as I am concerned, we should avoid them in favor of prescription migraine medications, whether for abortive use, preventive use, or both.

A migraine diagnosis generally does not need medical consultation, because it often suffices to look around and talk to family members. As mentioned, migraine is a genetically determined and inherited condition and, consequently, runs in families, affecting both men and women.

A misunderstanding is that it is a disorder exclusively concerning women. Men with migraine often suffer under the cover of bad tension headaches, bad sinus headaches, or bad hangover headaches, which do not exist. As a result, they deprive themselves of effective treatment, both abortively and preventively.

If the headaches are of relatively recent onset, starting weeks or months ago, especially if the patient is older, they warrant medical consultation to ascertain that a medical or neurological condition other than migraine does not cause them.

In this context, it is important to remember that headache intensity is not what matters in opposition to the significance physicians and other health care practitioners generally ascribe to "the worst headache ever." In fact, the worse the headache, the less likely medical or neurological illness other than migraine or a migraine-related disorder causes it.

This also means that even mild headaches can be of significance in terms of indicating medical or neurological illness. An example is the continuous, or persistent, low-grade headache that can be a symptom of hypothyroidism.

From a neurological perspective, a mild headache that was nothing more than a throbbing sensation in the right temple suggested to me a brain cause of mild clumsiness of the left hand. In this case, an abscess in the right half of the brain, called cerebral hemisphere, caused the clumsiness of the left hand and the throbbing in the right temple.

Brain function crosses over, which means that an abnormality in the right half of the brain, or cerebral hemisphere, causes problems in the left side of the body in terms of movement or feeling. However, pain is not crossed. As a result, with an abnormality in the right cerebral hemisphere, we feel pain, if present, in the right side of the head.

In terms of the intensity of the pain, it is important to realize that the brain itself is not sensitive to pain. If we feel pain, it is because the abnormality is big enough to affect structures surrounding it that are pain sensitive, such as the blood vessels on the surface of the brain that end up stretched as a result.

A lesson learned here is that we should never ignore headache, whatever its intensity, particularly if it is new, persistent, associated with other symptoms, or has changed in character.

Neurologist

With a complaint like headache, people tend to go to a neurologist, referred or not, but I do not recommend that. The reason is that neurologists generally do not consider the medical causes of headaches and focus on the neurological, brain-related ones only. However important this is, I nevertheless think that the initial consultation should be with a primary care physician, general practitioner, or family physician.

A diagnosis of migraine lies well within the realm of their competencies. Basic measurements like body temperature, pulse rate, and blood pressure can provide clues as to potential medical causes. Even a mildly elevated body temperature can point to an infection or autoimmune disorder as the cause of the headaches.

We should only attribute a low pulse rate to an excellent physical condition if there is indeed good reason to do so. Otherwise, we should look at it as potentially indicating low thyroid function, or hypothyroidism. Elevated blood pressure, we should never attribute to headache even if headache is present and severe, because it can easily be the cause of the headaches or worsening thereof.

The consulted physician or other health care practitioner should consider basic blood work, consisting of erythrocyte sedimentation rate (ESR), red and white blood cell count, ferritin, and thyroid function (thyroid-stimulating hormone, or TSH, and free levothyroxine level, or FT4).

Sedimentation rate and white blood cell count can provide further information regarding the possibility of infection or autoimmune disorder. Red blood cell count and ferritin can reveal anemia, iron deficiency, or both; along with thyroid function, it is important that they be considered, particularly if fatigue is an issue as well.

Consultation with a neurologist should happen only upon referral, and the same is true for consulting an eye specialist, also called ophthalmologist; or an ear, nose, and, throat specialist, or otolaryngologist.

It is important to remember that ophthalmologists generally have limited knowledge of headaches and otolaryngologists of face pain. Therefore, do not get disappointed when you see them for your headaches or face pain. They may not have the answer for you and, hence, no suggestions as to the treatment you are looking for to decrease your suffering and improve the quality of your life.

Chapter 4
What Is Migraine?

Inherited

Migraine is a genetically determined and inherited condition that runs in families. It is two to three times more common in women than in men; hence, first considering the women in the family makes sense.

As migraine is common and affects 15–20 percent of the population, looking at first-degree relatives—meaning parents, siblings, and children—generally suffices, although sometimes, it skips a generation. It is most common in the age group fifteen to forty-five, because it tends to get better as we get older, especially in women when they stop menstruating and become menopausal.

Men are notorious for not recognizing that they have migraine and may, instead, claim to suffer from bad tension headaches or bad sinus headaches. Sometimes, all they have is a history of bad hangover headaches when they were younger, causing them to stop drinking when they realize their intolerance to alcohol.

Most of the time, however, it is the mother who has migraine, but it is generally worse for the offspring when the father has it. The reason is that women develop migraine more easily than men do, because of the estrogen cycle related to the menstrual cycle, a very potent, if not the most potent, headache trigger.

Men obviously do not have this trigger and, consequently, have a higher genetic burden when they manifest migraine. They pass this higher burden on to their children, who consequently are more likely to develop it and also tend to do so at an earlier age, often already in childhood.

Migraine generally manifests itself between the ages of five and fifteen with a peak in girls in the early teens when they start menstruating. The first occurrence of menstruation we call menarche, and migraine typically develops within a year of it. If not then, women tend to manifest it during adolescence or early adulthood with the use of estrogen-containing birth control or in early to mid adulthood, related to pregnancy.

In relation to the latter, migraine more commonly develops after, rather than during, pregnancy, or after nursing when menstruation recurs. Often, not always, the ensuing headaches arise in relation to the menstrual cycle—that is, premenstrually in the days preceding menstruation, midcycle at the time of ovulation, or at the tail end of menstruation.

Birth Control

With a naturally occurring menstrual cycle, the worst headaches generally happen one or two days before menstruation, or premenstrually. With an artificial menstrual cycle—that is, the one created by the cyclical use of estrogen-containing birth control taken three weeks on and one week off—the worst headaches occur on the first day of the vaginal bleeding.

Women typically start cyclical estrogen-containing birth control on a Sunday with the bleeding and headache occurring on the Wednesday of the week off. Sometimes, people claim that this headache is not from the birth control, because it happens during the week off. This is faulty reasoning, because under those circumstances, estrogen withdrawal takes place and causes it.

If this is the case, it is important to discontinue the birth control immediately, because otherwise, there is a good chance that the headaches will continue to be a problem. In my experience, it may take as long as four to six months before the negative effect of estrogen-containing birth control on headaches wears off. Therefore, it is important not to draw conclusions hastily if the ultimate goal is to restart the birth control.

In general, I recommend that women avoid estrogen-containing birth control altogether because of its potential ill effects on health, not limited to headaches. There is also no longer a need to use this type of birth control because of the ubiquitous availability of birth control methods that contain the progestin component of estrogen-containing birth control only.

Estrogen-containing birth control, as the name implies, has an estrogen hormone in it, but it contains a progestin hormone as well. It is a so-called combination product with an estrogen and a progestin, the latter a form of the naturally occurring hormone progesterone, which plays an important role in the menstrual cycle and in pregnancy.

Progestins are synthetic hormones that we also refer to as progestogens, progestagens, gestogens, or gestagens. They mimic some of the effects of progesterone with the advantage that we can take them in tablet form by mouth.

Progesterone itself we can only take this way if it is micronized. Otherwise, we have to administer it as a vaginal gel or suppository, rectal suppository, or intramuscular injection. Physicians and other health care practitioners prescribe it in these formulations to prevent premature labor and not for birth control purposes.

In a combination estrogen-progestin birth control, the progestin works as birth control by thickening the mucus at the entry of the uterus, called cervix. This makes it impossible for sperm to penetrate the uterus and fertilize an egg released by the ovary. The estrogen has a cosmetic function only in the sense that it causes a vaginal bleeding to occur during the week off when the birth control is taken cyclically.

Sometimes, we use a combination estrogen-progestin birth control noncyclically, or continuously, which we generally do only when it contains a low dose estrogen—that is, ten to twenty micrograms per tablet. Physicians and other health care practitioners may recommend it for the treatment of menstrual migraine, which is migraine with the predominant occurrence of headaches around the time of menstruation, or perimenstrually. This may work due to the suppression of ovulation, but we need to monitor the overall frequency of headaches carefully, because it may increase.

Progestin-only Birth Control

Progestin-only birth control comes in several forms so that we can tailor it to a woman's need and preference. It comes in tablet form, often referred to as minipill, because it contains a progestin hormone only. The woman takes it daily without interruptions, and no vaginal bleedings happen, but sometimes, it causes spotting or breakthrough bleeding. A nonprescription birth control pill of this kind is available that contains seventy-five micrograms of the progestin, called norgestrel.

A formulation that has been around for several decades is an intramuscular depot injection that provides birth control for three months. A more recently developed one is an implant that we place into the skin, providing effective birth control for three years. The progestin-containing uterine inserts provide birth control for up to seven years and are generally easier to remove than the skin implant when desiring pregnancy. An insert like that is also referred to as an intrauterine system (IUS) and should not be confused with an intrauterine device (IUD).

Progestin-only birth control prevents menstruation, because it requires a drop in progesterone effect, which does not occur as long as progestin is in the body. It was not developed to suppress ovulation, but it does so nevertheless, although not consistently, in the majority of women, especially with prolonged use.

Suppression of ovulation means cessation of the estrogen cycle that accompanies the menstrual cycle; the estrogen cycle is what is generally detrimental to headache. Therefore, the use of progestin-only birth control can ameliorate migraine if the headaches happen predominantly related to the menstrual cycle—that is, premenstrually, midcycle at the time of ovulation, or at the tail end of menstruation. However, the indication should always be the need for highly effective birth control and never the management of migraine.

Menopause

What I wrote about avoiding estrogen-containing birth control altogether applies to menopausal estrogen therapy as well. Although its use has dramatically declined, physicians and other health care practitioners still prescribe it occasionally for the treatment of menopausal symptoms, particularly hot flashes and night sweats.

What they often fail to mention is that such treatment is merely postponement of execution, meaning that after discontinuation of the estrogen therapy, the complaints return unabated. I think that it is better to cope with them as best as possible and wait it out, knowing that they will ultimately improve, although this may take anywhere from months to years.

If we are dealing with severely disrupted sleep, we can use a medication, preferably trazodone, to treat the insomnia. The regular prescription sleeping medications, or hypnotics, make sleep dependent on them, rendering it difficult, if not impossible, to stop them.

Trazodone is officially an antidepressant, but it provides very little, if any, such benefit. Therefore, it is rarely, if ever, employed anymore for the treatment of depression. However, since the introduction of fluoxetine in the late 1980s, we have prescribed it extensively for insomnia.

Fluoxetine is a great antidepressant, but it can cause insomnia, and trazodone came in handy to treat the insomnia. It generally does not have side effects, particularly increased appetite and weight gain, often seen with psychiatric medications.

If trazodone causes daytime drowsiness, either the dose is too high, or the medication is used too late at night. The patient should take it at bedtime and preferably no later than ten or eleven o'clock. If falling asleep is also a problem, they can use it two hours earlier. Of course, one should not drive or operate machinery after taking it, because it causes drowsiness.

It is advisable to start with a low dose—for example, 25 milligrams—and increase it slowly until we achieve the nightly goal of eight or nine hours of uninterrupted sleep. If even the low dose of 25 milligrams causes daytime drowsiness, the patient can use 12.5 milligrams instead and can even take it at dinnertime as long as there is no driving afterward.

Trazodone does not make your sleep dependent on using it, which means that you can stop it anytime without repercussions, which is important. It works best for sleep when taken daily, and it requires approximately three days of consecutive use for maximum benefit.

Occasionally, I prescribe a medication called quetiapine for insomnia, especially if it is severe or when the patient also struggles with relentless anxiety. It is an antipsychotic with a strong antianxiety effect, but I use it in much lower dosages. The antipsychotic dose is 400–800 milligrams per day, while the one I use for insomnia lies usually between 12.5 and 50 milligrams per day, taken once daily at bedtime.

If the patient has problems falling sleep as well, which is often the case, they can use it two hours prior or at dinnertime. Of course, one should not drive or operate machinery after taking it, because it causes drowsiness.

Although the estrogen exposure with menopausal estrogen therapy is easily ten times lower than with estrogen-containing birth control, I have still seen the impact on headaches. Initially, we also prescribed it cyclically, as is customary with estrogen-containing birth control—that is, three weeks on and one week off. Under those circumstances, I saw headaches occur every time the patient started it or stopped it, confirming that estrogens can cause headaches upon exposure and withdrawal.

This, by the way, is similar to caffeine, which can also cause headaches upon exposure and withdrawal but, obviously, through a different mechanism. In both, the headaches from withdrawal are worse, sometimes much worse, than those caused by exposure.

Coming back to menopausal estrogen therapy, upon discontinuation, I have seen full resolution of migraine headaches, a menopausal benefit otherwise negated by the estrogen therapy.

Childhood

When migraine develops in early childhood, which happens because of a significant genetic burden—for example, when the father has migraine or a history thereof—it affects boys and girls equally often. The divergence in migraine occurrence between men and women does not happen until the early teens, when girls start menstruating.

In early childhood and when it comes to migraine, headache frequency and headache intensity are generally limited. The headaches tend to be sporadic and relatively mild. However, abdominal complaints are often abundantly present in terms of nausea, vomiting, and sometimes, also discomfort or pain.

When belly symptoms dominate the presentation, we refer to it as abdominal migraine, and headache can even be absent. It is a condition tricky to diagnose, however, and I have seen children and young adults with this diagnosis have their complaints resolved by treating their constipation.

Regarding the headaches, special attention is required if they are present on awakening in the morning in significant intensity or when they wake the child from sleep at night. Both scenarios are common in migraine, especially at an older age, but are ominous in childhood.

Then, they suggest the possibility of a brain tumor located in the back of the head, in the little brain or cerebellum. Such a brain tumor easily causes enlargement of the chambers in the brain, called ventricles. This leads to a disorder known as hydrocephalus, which manifests itself through severe headaches that develop overnight.

In terms of the treatment of headaches in children, I prefer to avoid pain medications, or analgesics, in early childhood. A good alternative under those circumstances is diphenhydramine, especially in its liquid formulation. It contains 12.5 milligrams of the medication per 5 milliliters and is easy to administer to a young child.

As it is already dissolved, it gets absorbed rapidly for fast relief. It soothes the stomach and, by doing so, relieves nausea and vomiting; in addition, it causes drowsiness, allowing the child to sleep. One of the characteristics of early-childhood migraine is that the headaches resolve with a nap; otherwise, relieving migraine headaches minimally requires overnight sleep.

Migraine Onset

In early childhood, migraine generally manifests itself spontaneously, as explained, due to a high genetic burden. In the early teens, girls often present with migraine within a year of menarche—that is, the onset of menstruation. In adolescence and early adulthood, the use of estrogen-containing birth control may cause the appearance of migraine. With the latter used cyclically, headaches typically occur in the week off due to estrogen withdrawal.

In men, alcohol exposure in early adulthood may cause the manifestation of migraine as bad hangover headaches. In women, in early to mid adulthood, pregnancy is quite commonly the reason migraine displays itself and much more so after than during pregnancy.

At any age, a head, neck, or back injury or stressful life event can cause migraine to ensue. Regarding the latter, in the same way as migraine headaches triggered by stress come afterward, during relaxation, the migraine can manifest itself post-stress here as well. The stressful life event can be good or bad in the same way as stress triggering a migraine headache can be good or bad.

Examples of stressful life events that can be associated with migraine manifestation are illness, surgery, moving, school, work, and marriage. Its appearance following gynecological surgery involving removal of the ovaries—for example, as part of a so-called total hysterectomy—can also be due to the postsurgical initiation of menopausal estrogen therapy.

Especially in adolescent boys, I have seen the onset of migraine related to the development of a delayed sleep phase disorder. This is a particular form of insomnia, very similar to a significant jet lag traveling east. It takes hours to fall asleep, it is impossible to get up in the morning, and it leaves you feeling exhausted all day. This is different with general insomnia, also referred to as primary insomnia, in which it is difficult to fall asleep, and frequent awakenings and early-morning awakenings shortcut sleep.

Insomnia

Of course, primary insomnia is also a condition associated with fatigue and, thus, a potential cause of headaches but often not to the extent that a delayed sleep phase disorder is. This may be because in delayed sleep phase disorder, the sleep is out of phase with the physiology of the body, which is not the case in primary insomnia.

In the latter, the interrupted sleep is generally more detrimental to energy buildup than the problems falling asleep and waking up early. In addition, its treatment is easier than that of a delayed sleep phase disorder, which sleeping medications, or hypnotics, tend to make worse. It concerns a disturbance of the biological clock, which is fortunately temporary in jet lag but is a continuing state here. As you can imagine, it interferes tremendously with daytime performance, whether at work or at school.

If moving west is not an option, finding a job with a three-to-eleven-o'clock shift can solve the problem, but that is obviously not feasible at school. By the time an adolescent with a delayed sleep phase disorder feels half decent, struggling with exhaustion and often with headache as well because of the insomnia, school is finished for the day. Homeschooling or home tutoring is generally the only possibility left, and understandably, it takes them a lot of effort to do well academically.

Delayed sleep phase disorder is treated with melatonin, a hormone that has an important function in the circadian rhythm, which is the twenty-four-hour internal clock, or sleep-wake cycle. It is crucial that the patient takes it daily in a very consistent manner, two hours before desired bedtime or sleep time. They should use it in an immediate-release formulation and not in a sustained-release one.

In the context of sleep, I would also like to mention insomnia due to restless legs syndrome, or RLS. It is a condition that mostly affects the ability to fall asleep because of a very uncomfortable feeling in the legs, associated with an irresistible urge to move them. Once it is possible to fall asleep, sleep is generally good without interruptions or early-morning awakening. The uncomfortable feeling in the legs can start upon lying down in bed to retire but can also already commence in the evening upon winding down.

Insomnia due to restless legs syndrome tends to respond poorly to general sleeping medications, or hypnotics; in my experience, a medication called pramipexole treats it best. It is marketed for the treatment of Parkinson's disease, but it very effectively treats restless legs syndrome as well. Patients generally tolerate it well without side effects, even with prolonged use, which is generally necessary.

Specifically for the treatment of restless legs syndrome, I prescribe it twice daily at dinnertime and at bedtime. Generally, a small dose, like 0.125 milligrams, taken at those times provides benefit; sometimes, a higher dose is required, such as 0.25 milligrams twice daily.

Chapter 5

How Does Migraine Manifest Itself?

Headache

The centerpiece of migraine in terms of its presentation is recurrent, intense headaches, which means headaches that are moderate or severe or have an intensity of at least a four on a ten-point scale. Indications of their being that intense are the lack of substantial relief by nonprescription pain medications, their association with nausea or vomiting, the need to suspend activity or lie down, and headaches waking the patient from sleep.

Slowed emptying of the stomach causes the lack of substantial relief by nonprescription pain medications as well as the association with nausea or vomiting. Once headaches escalate beyond a four on a ten-point scale, they activate the sympathetic nervous system to the extent that it retards stomach emptying.

The sympathetic nervous system is the part of the involuntary or autonomic nervous system that is stimulated by mental or physical stress. It makes our heart pound and gives us butterflies in the stomach. Headache is a physical stress that activates it as much as mental stress does, and the activation is directly proportional to the intensity of the pain.

The slowing of stomach emptying causes retention of its content, whatever it is, including any tablets or capsules taken to relieve the headache. Medications are not absorbed in the stomach but in the small bowel, and in order to get there, they must pass through the stomach—that is, the stomach needs to move them along.

During moderate or severe migraine headaches, the stomach does not pass medications along in the way it should, resulting in decreased efficacy. Generally, only medications that specifically address migraine headache can, through their potency, overcome this impact and, regardless, provide substantial relief. They do render better benefit, however, when taken at mild headache intensity or at an intensity of a four or less on the ten-point scale.

The goal of abortive migraine treatment is *full* relief of headache within two hours, and we can generally only accomplish this with a medication taken by mouth if taken at mild headache intensity. We can, of course, also administer it in other ways than by mouth or orally—that is, non-orally, such as by nasal spray, rectal suppository, or injection. The slowed stomach emptying does not affect their absorption if taken rectally or by injection. This is not necessarily the case, however, when administered by nasal spray, because the lining of the nose is not great at absorbing medications.

In addition, fluid nasal sprays have the problem that, due to their volume, medication drips out in the front and in the back. What drips out in the back subsequently makes its way to the stomach, passes through it, and gets absorbed in the small bowel.

For example, with the liquid triptan nasal sprays for abortive migraine treatment, as much as 70–85 percent of the medication drips down the back of the throat. Hence, with those sprays, most of the medication is absorbed in the small bowel rather than in the nose; consequently, its efficacy is affected by the slowed stomach emptying aforementioned.

This is less of an issue with powder nasal sprays, because powder medication sticks better to the lining of the nose than liquid medication, and in addition, there is less dripping in the front and in the back. Combining it with a so-called membrane permeability enhancer is another way of making the absorption of an intranasal medication less dependent on the stomach and, therefore, less dependent on headache intensity.

Nausea

Retention of stomach content is also the reason migraine headaches are associated with nausea but generally only when they are moderately severe or severe. When headaches of lesser intensity are associated with it, there is likely a stomach problem. If this is the case, it is important to identify what is wrong and treat it, because doing so may improve the headaches as well.

It is advisable to treat migraine-related nausea with medications that do not slow down stomach emptying any further. A simple antacid, such as calcium carbonate, may do the job, and medications like domperidone and metoclopramide may even improve stomach emptying.

We should avoid medications like prochlorperazine and ondansetron because, while treating nausea effectively, they further retard stomach emptying. We should certainly not combine them with oral medications to treat the headache, because it is already difficult enough for those to get absorbed the way it is.

We see vomiting only with the worst headaches, and the patient may throw up food ingested quite some time before. In early childhood, it may be associated with significant relief of the headache or termination thereof. Adults with migraine are not that fortunate although they may experience temporary reprieve afterward.

If possible, however, we should attempt to prevent vomiting, because the act itself is painful to the head when migraine headache is present. Antacids or medications like domperidone and metoclopramide are most beneficial here, because they do not impair stomach emptying and may even improve it. Patients generally tolerate them well without side effects, particularly fatigue or drowsiness.

Apart from gastrointestinal symptoms—particularly nausea, sometimes vomiting, and occasionally diarrhea—migraine headaches are associated with increased sensitivity of the senses. Sensitivity to light, also called photophobia, is generally the first to appear with escalating headache intensity, followed by sensitivity to noise, or phonophobia. With a further increase in headache intensity, nausea is likely to follow, along with sensitivity to smell, called osmophobia or odorphobia.

Only when the headache becomes very severe will vomiting occur, as mentioned, a point in headache escalation that we definitely want to avoid. Once a migraineur becomes that sick, we can only expect injectable treatment to provide relief, although if they are not averse to it, a rectal suppository may be helpful as well.

The one that makes sense to have in the refrigerator if headache does increase to the point of vomiting, no matter how rarely, is promethazine. As an antihistamine, it eases the stomach, potentially relieving nausea and vomiting, and is sedating, causing drowsiness. It is important to take a good dose, however—for example, fifty milligrams—and repeat it, if necessary, after an hour. Using this high a dose will likely cause drowsiness to the extent that sleep will follow, and when in a severe migraine headache, this is a blessing.

In this context, it is important to remember that apart from childhood migraine, which a nap may relieve, it generally takes overnight sleep to recover from a migraine headache. One may still wake up with residual headache the next day, however, especially if it has been present for days.

Emergency Room

Allowing a severe migraine headache with vomiting to continue may ultimately create a vicious cycle that is hard to break in any other way than through an emergency room visit. Such a visit involves treatment with intravenously administered medications, a scenario that we should avoid as well. Emergency rooms are full of hustle and bustle, brightly lit with fluorescent lights, and noisy with high-frequency beeps and chatter, making it the very last place in the world a migraineur wants to be in the midst of a severe headache.

The medications given intravenously for headache in an emergency room are not specific to migraine. Therefore, they may not provide more than temporary benefit, hopefully long enough, however, for the patient to get back home and go to sleep.

Common medications administered in this setting are ketorolac, an anti-inflammatory pain medication; hydromorphone, an opioid or narcotic pain medication; and ondansetron, prochlorperazine, promethazine, or metoclopramide as anti-nausea medications.

Regarding promethazine, we should never give it intravenously, because it can cause severe inflammation of the vein through which we administer it. When giving metoclopramide intravenously, we should always combine it with diphenhydramine to prevent restlessness, called akathisia, from occurring as a side effect.

Several of these medications, particularly diphenhydramine, hydromorphone, prochlorperazine, and promethazine, cause drowsiness. Consequently, we should not expect to return to normal functioning—for example, going back to work—after an emergency room visit.

Specific abortive migraine medications that we could give during emergency room visits for headache but hardly ever, if ever, do and for no good reason are sumatriptan and dihydroergotamine. Sumatriptan is available for subcutaneous injection under the skin in three dosages—three, four, and six milligrams—which we should repeat after an hour if well-tolerated and if it not fully relieved the headache.

The dose of dihydroergotamine is one milligram, administered subcutaneously or in the muscle after intramuscular injection of an anti-nausea medication, preferably one that does not cause drowsiness, such as metoclopramide or ondansetron. As mentioned, severe headaches are associated with nausea, if not with vomiting as well, and dihydroergotamine may aggravate those symptoms, especially if we do not provide an anti-nausea medication first.

While the subcutaneous administration of sumatriptan relieves severe headaches in twenty to forty minutes, dihydroergotamine easily takes one to two hours to do the same, but the relief potentially lasts much longer, often days. With sumatriptan, on the other hand, the headache may return in twelve to sixteen hours, sometimes so vigorously that it requires another injection for relief.

Sympathetic Nervous System

The associated complaints commonly encountered with migraine headaches, like nausea, vomiting, photophobia, phonophobia, and osmophobia, we often consider specific to migraine and employ them to diagnose the condition. As far as I am concerned, both are wrong; the symptoms are not specific to migraine, and we should not rely on them diagnostically, if only for the reason that they are not specific.

They are due to activation of the sympathetic nervous system, which is, as mentioned, the part of the involuntary or autonomic nervous system that makes our heart pound and gives us butterflies in the stomach. Pain stimulates the sympathetic nervous system, and there is plenty of it present in the setting of a migraine headache. The activation parallels the intensity of the headache, causing photophobia, followed by phonophobia, followed by nausea and osmophobia, and finally, leading to vomiting.

The abundant presence of sympathetic nervous system symptoms during migraine headaches suggests intense pain, maybe even more so than we generally realize, relatively low threshold for its activation, or both. Other complaints we commonly see with migraine headaches and of the same origin are paleness of the face, or pallor, and coldness of the nose, hands, and feet.

In terms of diagnosing migraine, we should focus on recurring headaches of high intensity, which as already explained we can deduce, among others, from the associated symptoms, but we should not exclusively rely on that.

There are certainly people with migraine who have the intense, recurring headaches characteristic of the condition but who do not have any of the aforementioned associated complaints. It is paramount that, in those patients, we also diagnose migraine so that they benefit as well from the medications specifically developed for the treatment of this so often debilitating disorder.

While headache intensity, as explained, is a feature of migraine in the sense that it is high, headache frequency is not. This means that you can have migraine and have headaches occasionally, maybe a couple of times per year or even less, or frequently, up to daily. When you have migraine headaches, it is something that you have in your genes, but having it in your genes does not explain the frequency in which you have them.

Muscle Tightness

Frequent migraine headaches are invariably associated with tight neck, shoulder, upper back, and often, jaw muscles as well. This muscle tightness is then probably also present in the head, but it is difficult to feel there, because there are no joints to move, as with the jaw and neck.

My impression is that under those circumstances, the muscle tightness drives the frequency of the headaches and may contribute to their intensity as well. I base this on my extensive experience with trigger point and botulinum toxin injections in headache patients, especially those with migraine.

We perform trigger point injections with a local anesthetic, like lidocaine, that we inject into tender spots in muscles, which we refer to as trigger points because pressure applied to them often results in pain felt remotely. An example is pressure exerted on a trigger point in the shoulder muscle causing pain in the temple on the same side. We know that injecting those spots with a local anesthetic relaxes the muscles, albeit temporarily; when we inject them with botulinum toxin, the benefit lasts much longer.

It is my experience that muscle injections with a local anesthetic or botulinum toxin can improve the frequency and intensity of migraine headaches. In fact, we have shown that thirty-one injections with botulinum toxin in the forehead, temples, back of the head, back of the neck, and shoulders benefit a migraine condition known as chronic migraine.

Chronic Migraine

Chronic migraine is a somewhat confusing term, because the adjective *chronic* has two meanings: “continuing for a long time” and "recurring frequently." Migraine is, by definition, a chronic condition in the sense that people suffer from it for years, if not decades. In the majority of cases, its onset is between the ages of five and fifteen, and it frequently does not abate until the age of fifty or sixty—in women, often related to the advent of menopause.

In the term *chronic migraine,* the adjective stands for recurring frequently, officially referring to a migraine disorder with a headache burden of half a month or more. Of course, in this definition, half a month or more is arbitrary, and there is nothing magical about it. Patients with chronic migraine generally have headaches daily or almost daily and, on average, have them well over twenty days per month.

Possibly a more meaningful way of defining chronic migraine is by considering it migraine that has lost its attack, or paroxysmal, pattern of headache occurrence. What characterizes migraine is recurring intense headaches, called attacks or paroxysms, that happen in well-defined episodes with distinct beginnings and distinct ends.

With increasing headache frequency, this attack or paroxysmal pattern is ultimately lost, resulting in the headaches blending into each other. This is something that, for sure, makes their abortive treatment more difficult and, therefore, may be a good reason to give it a different name.

When approached in this manner, it also makes sense to call the condition episodic if it has not reached the chronic stage because of the paroxysmal occurrence of the headaches. The half-a-month-or-more definition is suitable for clinical trial research, however, because of its operational nature. This is, indeed, what we initially intended it for and not for use in clinical practice, which unfortunately physicians and other health care practitioners often do not realize.

Comorbidities

From a medical perspective and probably more important than the episodic versus nonepisodic, or chronic, headache pattern is the general health of the patient. Apart from headaches, patients with episodic migraine are usually healthy while those with chronic migraine tend to have multiple medical and psychiatric conditions, which we commonly refer to as comorbidities.

We generally assume that comorbidities are disorders independent of the one they are associated with. However, when it comes to migraine, this may not be true, and I like to include them in my treatment, ultimately to the benefit of the migraine and the migraineur.

High on the list are the psychiatric conditions anxiety and depression, which are almost invariably present in patients with chronic migraine. Also common are fatigue and insomnia, both of which I do not consider psychiatric, although they are often viewed as such.

We will undoubtedly do better if we deem insomnia a neurological disorder and fatigue a metabolic one. Insomnia may well be the cause of fatigue, if present, but there may also be other reasons for the patient to feel tired, such as anemia, iron deficiency, or low thyroid function, that is hypothyroidism.

I already mentioned the invariable presence with chronic migraine of tightness of the neck, shoulder, upper back, and often, also of the jaw muscles. Muscle tightness like that, we generally assume, is the result of stress, but I think that when present continuously, or persistently, fatigue is more often the culprit. Fatigue means a lack of metabolic energy, and muscles need energy to relax; without it, they remain contracted and, hence, tight.

The above muscle tightness may also involve other postural muscles than the ones mentioned, particularly the lower-back muscles and calf muscles. When the tightness affects the latter, it may manifest itself in leg or foot cramps, called charley horses after an old horse Charley, or in a condition referred to as restless legs syndrome, or RLS.

Charley horses happen during exercise but are especially troublesome when they occur at night, causing awakening from sleep in severe pain. Treatment with thiamine, or vitamin B_1, one hundred milligrams per day, I have found helpful for the prevention of those painful cramps.

Restless legs syndrome is a particular cause of insomnia, characterized by problems falling asleep due to an irresistible urge to move the legs. Its most effective treatment is with a medication for Parkinson's disease called pramipexole, taken at dinnertime and at bedtime.

Sometimes, the muscle tightness extends from the core of the body, the trunk, into the extremities, and then we refer to it as fibromyalgia.

Due to the muscles of the digestive tract getting involved, stomach and large-bowel disorders are also quite common comorbidities of chronic migraine. If the stomach does not empty out well on a regular basis, acid retention may lead to complaints like heartburn, reflux, nausea, or stomach pain.

If not emptying out well regularly is the case with the large bowel, constipation develops with infrequent bowel movements and hard stool that is difficult to evacuate. The constipation, in turn, may lead to diarrhea, which in this context is referred to as paradoxical diarrhea, and the condition, subsequently, may evolve into irritable bowel syndrome of the mixed type.

Irritable bowel syndrome, or IBS, comes in three presentations: constipation-predominant, or IBS-C; diarrhea-predominant, or IBS-D; and mixed, or IBS-M. We diagnose it when an abnormal bowel movement pattern is associated with abdominal discomfort or pain, typically relieved by a bowel movement or movements.

General Population

Approximately 20 percent of those who have migraine—that is, one out of five migraineurs—have headaches frequently enough to qualify for the diagnosis chronic migraine. In those patients, we determine the total headache burden based on the number of days with migraine but also on the days with other headaches, such as tension headache or sinus headache.

In migraineurs, headaches in general, whether tension or sinus, quickly progress to migraine headaches and become moderate or severe in intensity. As migraine affects approximately 15 percent of the general population, it means that approximately 3 percent has chronic migraine, which is quite a significant number.

Approximately the same percentage has daily or almost daily headaches of mild intensity without intense migraine headaches. We refer to this headache presentation as chronic muscle contraction headache, chronic tension headache, or chronic tension-type headache. People generally do not seek medical consultation for it, because nonprescription pain medications relieve the headaches, at least temporarily, which is not the case with migraine.

Of the approximately 12 percent of migraineurs in the general population with episodic migraine, the majority has migraine without aura, which we used to call common migraine. This migraine condition affects approximately 10 percent of the population, and the remaining 2 percent has migraine with aura, which we previously referred to as classic migraine.

Considering it from a general population perspective, approximately 10 percent has migraine without aura, approximately 2 percent has migraine with aura, and approximately 3 percent has chronic migraine.

Migraine without aura and migraine with aura are the two most common presentations of episodic migraine. The difference is that in migraine with aura, an aura precedes the headaches as a warning. It is usually visual in nature, affecting eyesight, and generally happens before the onset of the headache or during the initial phase of headache development.

Chapter 6

Why Do I Lose My Vision?

Visual Aura

In the context of migraine, you do not lose your vision, but a primitive hallucination may obscure it temporarily. This is what typically happens in migraine with aura, either before the onset of the headache or during the initial phase of headache development.

Abnormal activity in the back of the brain, in the so-called occipital cortex, where vision is located, is the culprit. It gives the impression that we are seeing something that, actually, is not there and, thus, accounts for the hallucination. However, we are not seeing anything complex, like a face or a person, but simple structures, like zigzag lines or spots. Hence, I refer to it as a primitive hallucination.

As it involves activation of the occipital cortex, the simple structures that we see are bright or flickering and sometimes colorful. In addition, the activity travels over the occipital cortex in a certain way, which makes the lines or spots move as well. The patient vignette below illustrates the rate at which it travels, causing the visual migraine aura typically to last fifteen to thirty minutes.

A forty-seven-year-old woman has been experiencing migraine since the age of nineteen. The headaches have gradually increased in frequency to once or twice per week. They generally come on during the day, build to their maximum intensity in two hours, and last one to three days.

The headaches are always located on the right and extend from the forehead, over the top of the head, into the back of the head. They are moderate or severe in intensity, throbbing in nature, and associated with light sensitivity and, when severe, with nausea as well. Two to four times per year, a visual disturbance precedes the headaches with a five- to ten-minute interval.

Over a four-year period, the patient had the visual disturbance thirteen times, of which six occurred on the left and seven on the right, all followed by right-sided headache. Three times, it started during sleep and was present on awakening in the morning. On ten occasions, it came on during the day, allowing her to time it from beginning to end.

The average duration of those ten visual disturbances was 25.2 minutes, ranging from 22 to 29 minutes. They consisted of an arch of wavy, zigzag lines, which gradually enlarged as the disturbance moved outward, followed by gray swirling as an afterimage. In addition, there were spots of missing vision that appeared before, during, or after the arch of wavy, zigzag lines.

We used to think that a narrowing of blood vessels, or vasoconstriction, in the back of the brain caused the visual migraine aura by depriving it of oxygen. We now know, however, that this is not the case and that a particular kind of activation of the visual part of the brain is the culprit.

The activation itself is short lasting, and a longer-lasting depression follows it. As we discovered the depression first because of its longer duration, we refer to it as spreading cortical depression while it is, in fact, spreading cortical excitation. We do not know what initiates it, why it happens, or what its purpose is. What we do know is that visual stimulation can bring on the visual migraine aura and that this is more likely to happen under circumstances of fatigue.

A typical scenario is driving on a road lined with trees in the spring or in the fall when the sun stands low, generating the kind of strobe-like stimulation that easily triggers a visual migraine aura. However, this is much more likely to happen in the evening—for example, while driving home from work—than in the morning, driving to work. The difference is that in the evening, especially after a day at work, we are tired, as opposed to in the morning, when rested after a night's sleep.

We apply this knowledge in the laboratory when we want to investigate the visual migraine aura. For the purpose of a study, we have the migraineur exercise vigorously—for example, by playing basketball—and then stimulate them visually in a strobe-like fashion.

Brain cells and muscle cells share the need for energy to undo their activity, which for muscle cells means relaxation. In a similar way, brain cells need energy to relax, although their relaxation, of course, does not go beyond undoing their activity.

If they do not quiet down, brain cells remain active and excitable and may even lapse into a seizure. This is something that can happen when pulling an all-nighter, as we encounter in college students who are up all night studying or recruits who stand guard all night.

Spreading cortical excitation may be the brain's safety valve to undo its activity when it is not able to do so naturally—for example, due to a lack of metabolic energy. Causing the primitive visual hallucination of the migraine aura and temporarily obscuring vision certainly beats falling down in a seizure!

The first sign of the visual presentation of the migraine aura is typically a twinkling spot near the center of vision. As the spot gradually enlarges, it opens up on the inside to give rise to a crescent or half-moon of flickering, zigzag lines that are bright and sometimes colorful. The crescent, which is called scintillating scotoma, fortification spectra, or teichopsia, subsequently slowly expands as it moves toward the periphery of the visual field in which it advanced.

The development of the visual migraine aura is usually in one visual field or the other, although very rarely it advances in both at the same time. Then it really becomes difficult to see and hazardous to drive. Driving with a migraine aura in just one visual field is already bad enough!

From start to finish, the visual migraine aura generally lasts fifteen to thirty minutes. It ends by fading away in the periphery of the visual field in which it developed or by moving outside the realm of vision.

Somatosensory Aura

It is possible for spreading cortical excitation to affect other areas of the brain than the occipital cortex, where vision is located. It is rare, however, that this happens and the symptoms that emerge are dependent on where in the brain the excitation occurs. The second most common place is the so-called somatosensory cortex in the side of the brain. This is where the brain receives and processes sensory information, such as touch, coming from the other side of the body, or soma. In the brain, everything is crossed, and the visual cortex in the back of the brain is no exception.

Activation of the somatosensory cortex causes a sensation of tingling in the opposite side of the body, similar to what we feel when a limb falls asleep. It may also give us the impression of weakness, akin to what we experience when we try to use a limb that has fallen asleep. We call this presentation resulting from activation of the somatosensory cortex cheiro-oral syndrome or digitolingual paresthesias.

It consists of tingling, generally commencing in the fingers of one hand, gradually moving up the arm, and ultimately affecting the nose-mouth area on the same side. An example of it follows in the patient vignette below, which also illustrates the third and least common migraine aura symptom, a speech problem due to involvement of the brain's speech center.

The visual aura in the patient vignette demonstrates the excitation component of the spreading cortical excitation-depression phenomenon in the crescent of flickering, zigzag lines. It shows the depression component in the grayness moving along with it as a band lying against its inside.

A thirty-five-year-old woman has been experiencing migraine since the age of nine. The headaches happen once or twice per year, preceded by a visual disturbance that consists of an area of grayness in the center of vision. On the right of the grayness, a crescent of flickering, zigzag lines develops, which gradually expands toward the periphery of the right visual field. As the crescent moves across the visual field, the grayness moves along with it as a band lying against its inside.

The visual disturbance lasts an hour, and headache follows it immediately. The headaches are located in the temple, usually on the right but sometimes on the left. They are severe, steady in nature and associated with nausea and, occasionally, with vomiting. The headaches last thirty-six hours. Going without food too long, strong odors, and exercise bring them on.

When the patient was on estrogen-containing birth control, the visual disturbance was associated with a feeling of tingling. It started in the fingers of the left hand and gradually extended upward into the forearm, ultimately skipping to the left side of the face, affecting the nose, mouth, tongue, and roof of the mouth. On one occasion and along with the visual disturbance, she experienced slurred speech and difficulty forming words.

In the above patient vignette and while on estrogen-containing birth control, the migraine aura expanded from impacting vision only to also including somatosensation and speech. The use of estrogen-containing birth control is associated with an increased risk of stroke, although minimally; the same is true, by the way, for menopausal estrogen therapy. However, we should not interpret the above change in aura presentation as stroke related; it is due to an effect of estrogens on energy metabolism instead.

Estrogens increase the binding of the thyroid hormones to the proteins in the blood, thereby preventing the hormones from entering the cells and doing their job. If the thyroid gland does not have the reserve capacity to compensate for this increased binding, it results in a lowering of thyroid function and, thus, of energy metabolism. This affects brain cell function in the sense that it hampers them, undoing their activity.

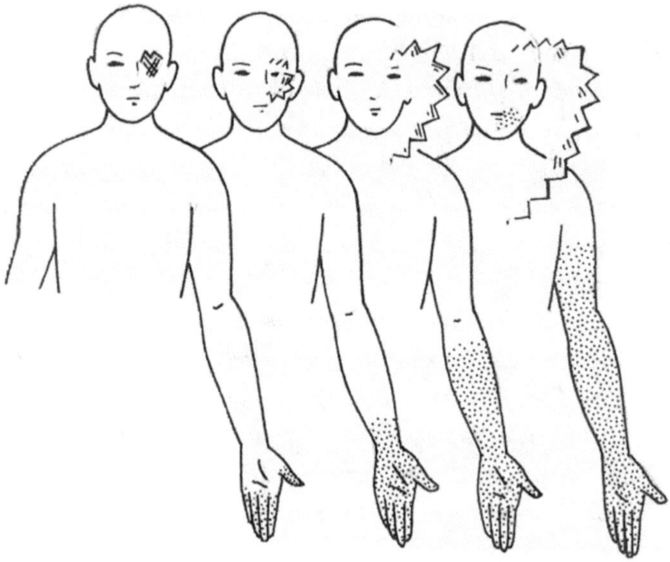

From left to right, a schematic presentation depicting the development of the visual migraine aura known as scintillating scotoma (upper) and of the somatosensory migraine aura known as digitolingual paresthesias (lower)

Chapter 7

What Causes the Pain in My Head?

Throbbing

Humanity has known migraine as a condition of recurring intense headaches for at least five thousand years with its first description reported to have appeared in 3,000 BC. Over history, the throbbing nature of migraine headaches has led people to think that a widening of blood vessels in the brain causes them.

The belief that cerebral vasodilation, which is what we call it, is the pain mechanism underlying migraine headaches persisted into the beginning of the last century. It became the subject of extensive investigation by a young neurologist from New York City, Harold G. Wolff, himself a migraineur.

In the 1920s, Professor Wolff came to Boston, Massachusetts, which in those days was at the forefront of clinical neurology and neurological research, to investigate brain blood flow in relation to migraine. Harvard scientists at Boston City Hospital, now Boston Medical Center, and Massachusetts General Hospital were studying brain blood flow, also referred to as cerebral circulation.

Professor Wolff, a researcher at heart and driven by an inquisitive mind, came to Boston to provide the scientific evidence for the understanding that migraine headaches are due to a widening of blood vessels in the brain. He intended to do so by means of a medication called ergotamine.

Ergotamine

The scientist and pharmacologist Professor Arthur Stoll isolated ergotamine at Sandoz Laboratories in Basel, Switzerland, in 1918. Sandoz Pharmaceuticals subsequently marketed it in the Unites States in 1921 under the brand name Gynergen, reflecting its gynecological indication, which was to stop heavy bleeding after childbirth, so-called postpartum hemorrhage, a leading cause of maternal death.

The indication for this particular use came from the fact that ergotamine potently contracted the womb, or uterus. However, physicians also knew that it potently contracted blood vessels—in its extreme, as evidenced by tissue death—called gangrene, especially in the fingers and toes. This happened in Europe during medieval times from eating bread baked with rye contaminated by the fungus Claviceps purpurea. It was from this fungus that Professor Stoll isolated ergotamine and advanced it as treatment for postpartum hemorrhage.

The belief that cerebral vasodilation was the underlying mechanism of the migraine headache quickly led to ergotamine's off-label use for abortive migraine treatment. What made it particularly valuable for migraine research was the fact that it was not a pain medication; it potently relieved migraine headaches while not relieving pain from other causes.

Professor Wolff's trip to Boston was disappointing, however, because the research did not reveal what he had expected. Ergotamine moderately increased brain blood flow, suggesting the opening rather than narrowing of blood vessels, or vasodilation rather than the expected vasoconstriction. In agreement, it also increased cerebrospinal fluid, or CSF, pressure, which is the pressure of the fluid in and around the brain and spinal cord.

The skull is a confined space, and the pressure within it increases when anything inside it takes more space—in this case, the volume of blood due to vasodilation. When the pressure inside the skull increases, so does the cerebrospinal fluid pressure, altogether providing double evidence that ergotamine widens rather than narrows the blood vessels of the brain.

Undoubtedly, Professor Wolff was greatly puzzled as to how the medication relieved migraine headaches if it further opened brain blood vessels that were already dilated to cause the migraine headache. He pursued this contradictory finding when my mentor in headache management, John R. Graham, joined him as his first assistant at New York Hospital, Cornell Medical School, in New York City.

They probably knew each other from Professor Wolff's time in Boston, because both were graduates of Harvard Medical School, and Professor Graham trained in internal medicine at Massachusetts General Hospital. He was also involved in the headache clinic at the hospital, which was probably the first of its kind in the United States, if not in the world.

Blood Vessels

Returning to the generally throbbing nature of migraine headaches and the blood vessels in the head, we divide those into three compartments. The first compartment is that of the brain blood vessels, which constitute the cerebral circulation. The second is that of the blood vessels on the outside of the brain but inside the skull, which are the meningeal, or dural, blood vessels. The third comprises the blood vessels on the outside of the skull—that is, in the scalp—which we refer to as the extracranial blood vessels.

If ergotamine does not constrict the blood vessels of the brain to relieve migraine headaches, Professors Graham and Wolff asked themselves the obvious question: What is its effect on the other blood vessels in the head?

The most accessible to study, of course, are the blood vessels on the outside of the skull, in the scalp, which are the extracranial ones. The most prominent of these is the superficial temporal artery, which runs from the ear, through the temple, to the forehead. You can feel it when you put the tip of a finger on the cheekbone just before the ear and exert a little pressure.

You can feel it throbbing with the heartbeat, because it is an artery, which is a blood vessel that carries oxygenated blood from the heart to the tissues in the body. You can sometimes see it where the temple transitions into the forehead, the so-called frontotemporal area.

When it is visible there, we often erroneously call it a vein, which is a blood vessel that returns blood from the tissues in the body to the heart. However, it is not a vein but an artery, and you can tell because it throbs with the heartbeat when you put your finger on it.

In their investigation, Professors Wolff and Graham put simple tambour devices on the superficial temporal artery as well as on other extracranial arteries, registering in this way the magnitude of their throbbing, the so-called pulsation amplitude. They did so in migraine patients in the midst of severe migraine headaches and administered the ergotamine intravenously to relieve their headaches, which happened within minutes.

Tracking the headache relief provided by the medication, they observed a strong reduction in the pulsation amplitude of the arteries. Thus, in contrast to the brain blood vessels, which widened, or dilated, in response to ergotamine, the extracranial blood vessels narrowed, or constricted. In fact, they constricted strongly and the constriction paralleled the rapid decrease in headache intensity that occurred.

As you can imagine, the meningeal or dural blood vessels that reside outside the brain but inside the skull were much more difficult to investigate. In order to study their response to ergotamine, Professors Graham and Wolff collaborated with the neurosurgeons at New York Hospital.

While patients were undergoing brain surgery and their skulls were opened, they measured the diameter of the middle meningeal artery, the biggest of the meningeal, or dural, blood vessels. These patients did not have migraine and were under general anesthesia, so consequently, there was no headache intensity to record. What they observed was a small reduction in diameter, indicating a vasoconstrictor effect, but by far not as pronounced as that of the extracranial arteries.

Due to the significance of the potential shift that resulted from the above experiments in understanding the location of the vasodilation of the migraine headache, Professor Wolff conducted another series of investigations in migraineurs. He studied them again during severe migraine headaches, but instead of giving them ergotamine to relieve their headaches, he performed lumbar punctures and raised their cerebrospinal fluid, or CSF, pressure by injecting saline, in this way dampening the throbbing of the cerebral *and* meningeal, or dural, blood vessels.

He observed that this procedure did not alleviate their headaches, supporting the developing understanding that extracranial vasodilation rather than cerebral or meningeal vasodilation causes the migraine headache. As a corollary, a medication like ergotamine relieves migraine headaches by constricting extracranial arteries; not by constricting cerebral or meningeal arteries.

Inflammation

Professor Wolff continued his quest to understand the mechanism behind the migraine headache by studying the sensitivity to pain of the extracranial arteries, again collaborating with the neurosurgeons. Patients who were undergoing brain surgery had their heads shaved, which made it easy to identify the superficial temporal artery as it runs from the ear, through the temple, to the forehead.

Before opening the skull for brain surgery, Professor Wolff placed a pair of medical pliers, called forceps, in the artery, which he subsequently distended by widening them. He inserted the pliers under local anesthesia and tested the painfulness of the arteries after the anesthesia had worn off. The patients reported the mechanical dilation, or distention, to be painful, but it was by far not enough pain to account for the intensity of the migraine headache. This convinced him that vasodilation alone could not explain migraine headaches, certainly not in terms of their intensity.

He subsequently wondered whether a decrease in pain threshold made the vasodilation painful enough. In order to investigate this, he studied migraine patients during and between migraine headaches and measured the pain threshold with a device called dolorimeter, or algometer.

Using this device, he exerted pressure on different spots in the frontotemporal area where the forehead meets the temple and where, if visible, we can see the superficial temporal artery. He observed that the deep pain threshold in the area of the pain was three times lower, on average, during migraine headaches than in between, confirming his suspicion.

What was the cause of the decrease in pain threshold at the site of the pain during migraine headache? Of course, this was the next question that emerged; in order to answer it, Professor Wolff conducted a more invasive experiment, again in migraine patients during and between migraine headaches.

He inserted two needles at some distance from each other in the frontotemporal area on the side of the headache, pushed saline in through one, and collected it from the other. From the tissue perfusion samples thus collected, he determined the inflammatory activity and found it to be high during severe migraine headaches. It was still high, but much less so during moderate headaches and afterward when the area was still tender, all in comparison to when no headache was present.

Vascular Theory

Based on the aforementioned and other investigations performed by Professor Wolff over the course of three decades and with the help of a dozen or more assistants, he arrived at the following understanding of what causes the migraine headache: A dilation of extracranial arteries stretches the pain nerve fibers that coil around them, thereby activating the nerve fibers to the extent that they fire off signals to the brain, resulting in the perception of pain.

At the same time, the nerve fibers release chemicals around the arteries that cause them to become inflamed, rendering them more sensitive to pain and, at the same time, widening them even further. In this way, a vicious cycle is set into motion, going downhill like an avalanche, rapidly progressing to severe headache, with the affected arteries dilated as well as inflamed.

We have come to refer to this explanation of migraine headache pathogenesis, as we call it, as the vascular theory of migraine. However, Professor Wolff probably also realized that in the context of migraine headache mechanism, the inflammation is much more important than the vasodilation. After all, vasodilation is merely blood vessel widening while inflammation is that *and* pain sensitization, or lowering of the pain threshold, making the vasodilation much more painful than it would be otherwise.

The inflammation involved in migraine is of a particular kind that we never really studied well in medicine and, consequently, know rather little about. We generally research inflammation in relation to infection—viral, bacterial, or fungal—degeneration, such as in osteoarthritis, or in the context of autoimmune diseases, such as Hashimoto's disease of the thyroid gland.

The inflammation of migraine is of a very different origin and comes from the activation of nerve fibers in the body that are particularly sensitive to painful stimulation, the so-called nociceptive nerve fibers. As it originates from the activation of nerve fibers, we call it neurogenic inflammation, with *neuro* indicating that it is related to nerves or to the nervous system.

Neurogenic inflammation involves a variety of chemicals that those nerve fibers release in the tissues affected, of which the best known are the so-called neuropeptides calcitonin gene-related peptide, or CGRP, neurokinin A, and substance P.

As to what causes the initial vasodilation, setting it all into motion by activating the mechanism of neurogenic inflammation, Professor Wolff had a hard time explaining. Consequently, he fell back, at least to a certain extent, to the old thinking and original beliefs. Although he had shown that cerebral vasodilation was not the underlying mechanism of the migraine headache, he was still convinced that it played a role and suggested that the extracranial vasodilation happened because of it.

However, there is no evidence that the two blood vessel systems of the head, cerebral and extracranial, which reside in different anatomical compartments, connect to each other in a functional way. This is also not plausible, because they serve entirely different purposes, with the circulation of the brain entirely subservient to and, hence, determined by brain activity to support it with the necessary oxygen and nutrients. The extracranial circulation, on the other hand, provides oxygen and nutrients to the head muscles and to the scalp and is involved in the body's temperature regulation as well.

Migraine Aura

If cerebral vasodilation happens with migraine headaches—and from brain blood flow studies conducted much later, we know that it does—the obvious question is why. In order to investigate this, Professor Wolff turned to the subgroup of migraineurs, approximately 15 percent of them, who have so-called migraine with visual aura.

These patients experience visual symptoms before the onset of their headaches or during the initial phase of headache development. Consequently, they definitely have something going on in their brain or, more precisely, in the back of their brain, where vision is located, just before or during the onset of a migraine headache. It is difficult to study migraine aura, however, because its occurrence is hard to predict, and it lasts only fifteen to thirty minutes, although occasionally longer, when we refer to it as migraine aura status.

Nevertheless, Professor Wolff succeeded in studying several patients during a visual migraine aura, and while documenting the progression of their auras, he treated them with amyl nitrate or carbon dioxide. Both are inhaled medications that work fast and were known to him from his prior research on cerebral circulation in Boston to widen, or dilate, brain blood vessels.

Amyl nitrate is similar to the nitroglycerine we prescribe for the treatment of angina of the heart—that is, chest pain upon exertion, often extending into the jaw or left arm, due to partial blockage of an artery of the heart.

With both treatments, he observed an improvement, or regression, of the aura symptoms, suggesting to him that a temporary blockage of blood flow to the part of the brain where vision is located caused them.

There is a neurological condition known as transient ischemic attack, or TIA, caused by just that—a temporary blockage of blood flow to a part of the brain. Depending on the part involved, it results in one-sided face drooping, one-sided arm weakness or numbness, one-sided loss of vision, or difficulty speaking, generally not lasting longer than a half hour or so.

We refer to it as a mini stroke or mini brain attack, and it is important to recognize it as such, because it may lead to a stroke with permanent symptoms, often resulting in significant disability. It can happen in an eye as well, referred to as amaurosis fugax, with similar duration. A quickly dissolving blood clot causes the temporary blockage in transient ischemic attack while a permanent clot causes a stroke or brain attack.

Amaurosis fugax is, however, very different in its presentation from the visual migraine aura in the sense that there is loss of vision in one eye as opposed to a primitive visual hallucination on one side of vision. The visual disturbance of migraine happens in both eyes but generally on one side of vision only, or in one visual field, which can be left or right.

Blood Vessel Spasm

As an astute neurologist, Professor Wolff was well aware of the differences in presentation between amaurosis fugax, or transient ischemic attack in general, and the visual migraine aura. Nonetheless and probably because he lacked a reasonable alternative, he thought that the underlying mechanism was the same in both—namely, a temporary interruption of blood flow—with the difference that in migraine it occurred due to blood vessel spasm rather than from a rapidly dissolving blood clot.

He subsequently proposed that the lack of oxygen due to the temporary blood vessel spasm caused the brain to respond by throwing its blood vessels open. Extracranial vasodilation, he suggested, was the accompaniment of this general cerebral vasodilation, setting into motion the vicious migraine headache cycle by initiating the mechanism of neurogenic inflammation.

This was the inflammation to which he had attributed the decrease in pain threshold at the site of the pain during migraine headache and the sensitivity of the blood vessels. However, what about the approximately 85 percent of migraineurs who do not experience aura with their headaches and have migraine without aura, as we now call it, which we used to refer to as common migraine?

Professor Wolff was a smart and ingenious man; no question was beyond his intellectual capability, whether he could research it or not. He proposed that when an aura was not present, the temporary blood vessel spasm still happened, but in an area of the brain where it did not cause symptoms, a so-called clinically silent area. By making this suggestion, he rendered the sequence of events leading to the migraine headache independent of whether an aura was present or not.

Migraine had traditionally only been considered as such if an aura was present, and similar headaches without aura were called sick headache, because they were generally associated with nausea, if not with vomiting as well. It was the contribution of American medicine that we also included sick headache in the migraine paradigm, initially named common migraine but now called migraine without aura.

Half a century or so later, the same happened with mixed or combined headache, a presentation of chronic tension headache brought under the migraine umbrella as chronic migraine. This was not a contribution of American medicine, however, but of American psychology, with the realization that approximately half of those with chronic tension headache had intense headaches similar to migraine.

The headaches responded abortively and preventively to migraine medications, and our consideration of them as migraine greatly improved the treatment of those patients. They came under the care of psychologists, because we used to deem chronic tension headache a depression equivalent, which meant depression presenting with continuous, low-grade headache rather than with feeling down in mood.

Brain Function

Regarding the visual migraine aura, we now know from much later studies, also conducted at Harvard Medical School, that it is caused by a disturbance in brain function rather than by a temporary blood vessel spasm. This disturbance consists of a spreading excitation of short duration, followed by a longer-lasting depression. An increase in brain blood flow accompanies the excitation while a decrease comes along with the depression, reflecting what I stated earlier, namely that brain blood flow serves brain metabolism and, consequently, mirrors brain activity.

Danish studies have shown increased brain blood flow with fully developed migraine headaches, undoubtedly due to the intense pain stimulating the brain, resulting in heightened brain activity and, consequently, increased brain circulation.

Pain in general activates the brain by stimulating the sympathetic nervous system, which is part of the involuntary or autonomic nervous system. Such activation is very prominent in migraine, resulting in symptoms like paleness of the face, or pallor, and coldness of the extremities, both due to vasoconstriction, and nausea and vomiting due to impaired stomach emptying.

The increased sensitivity of the senses, as in photophobia, phonophobia, and osmophobia—that is, light, noise, and smell sensitivity respectively—could result from the heightened arousal as well, also caused by the stimulation of the sympathetic nervous system.

Photophobia, or light sensitivity, however, can also have another explanation that is not related to the brain, as suggested by its association, at times, with blurred vision. Blurred vision does not originate from the brain and, therefore, is never an aura symptom; when it occurs with migraine headaches, we should consider it an associated complaint, similar to how we view photophobia or nausea.

Although we typically employ these associated symptoms to diagnose the condition, we have to keep in mind that they are not specific to migraine. We can see them in any situation in which the sympathetic nervous system is vigorously activated, migraine being only one of them.

Blurred Vision

If blurred vision precedes the onset of the headache like a prodrome, it indicates that eyestrain causes the migraine headache. The same applies, although to a somewhat lesser extent, to photophobia, or light sensitivity, happening before the onset of the headache.

Relevant to eyestrain, little muscles called muscles of accommodation, or ciliary muscles, surround the lenses in our eyes. When these muscles tighten, or contract, they make the lenses rounder, allowing us to see up close and helping our eyes cope with bright light. The ciliary muscles are so-called smooth muscles and as such have nerve fibers running through them, including specific ones that relax them. These relaxing nerve fibers are part of the sympathetic nervous system and get activated when the sympathetic nervous system is stimulated.

Relaxation of the ciliary muscles flattens the lenses, and this, in turn, results in photophobia, or light sensitivity, and, when pronounced, in blurred vision. Eyestrain does very much the same—not by stimulating the sympathetic nervous system, however, but by exhausting the muscles. In the process of eyestrain, headache can develop; if this happens in a migraineur, migraine headache is the result.

The same stresses or strains, mental or physical, bring on migraine headaches, as they bring on headaches in general, and whether the headache that ensues is a migraine headache or not depends on the vulnerability of the person. It is a specific vulnerability that we inherit, and that, I think, resides in the activation threshold of the aforementioned mechanism of neurogenic inflammation. The lower its threshold, the easier it is to bring on migraine headaches and the worse they are in terms of their intensity.

The intensity, in turn, drives the subsequent activation of the sympathetic nervous system and, consequently, the involvement of the body as a whole with resulting symptoms such as nausea, photophobia, and phonophobia. In addition, it determines, at least to some extent, the duration of the headaches, because the more intense they are, the longer the body requires to recover from them.

Usually, although not always, overnight sleep relieves migraine headaches, but they also commonly linger into the next day. Headaches that occur in relation to the menstrual cycle last even longer, often days, because they generally do not resolve until the underlying hormonal change levels off.

Connection

If the mechanisms underlying the migraine aura and migraine headache do not connect with each other in the way Professor Wolff suggested, which is through cerebral vasospasm, cerebral vasodilation, and extracranial vasodilation, do they connect at all? And if so, how?

As mentioned, there is no evidence that cerebral vasospasm, which is blood vessel spasm in the brain, happens in migraine without aura or for the occurrence here of the spreading excitation-depression phenomenon of the migraine aura. Furthermore, decreased blood flow is the ultimate result of the excitation-depression phenomenon and not cerebral vasodilation. Finally, there is no evidence that extracranial vasodilation accompanies cerebral vasodilation.

Overall, these are more than enough reasons, I assume, to abandon Professor Wolff's thinking of how migraine headaches, with or without aura, develop. However, we do not want to throw the baby out with the bathwater and should not lose sight of the fact that solid experimental investigations conducted in migraineurs constitute the basis of our extracranial vasodilation/inflammation understanding of migraine headache pathogenesis.

Concerning the migraine aura-headache connection, my opinion is that the migraine aura does not connect to the migraine headache in a cause-effect, or causal, manner as Professor Wolff proposed. Although I have been extensively involved in migraine research, I consider myself primarily a clinician and mostly base my thinking on clinical findings. Reflecting on the migraine aura-headache connection, the following observations, relevant to this topic, come to mind.

First, an aura only precedes the minority of migraine headaches, merely 10–15 percent. Second, headache does not always follow the aura, which may be more common than we generally surmise. Third, the aura and headache may happen with an overlap, simultaneously, or with a considerable time interval. Fourth and important from a brain perspective, the headache does not always occur on the opposite side of the aura; in fact, it may be on the same side or on both sides.

In context of the latter, it is important to remember that everything in the brain is crossed, except pain. This means that when, for example, something affects the right side of the brain that causes pain, the resulting symptoms will be on the left, except the pain—in this case, headache—which will be on the right.

My thinking regarding the migraine aura-headache connection is that in the migraine process, the brain gets involved in some but not in most patients and that it is *not* essential to the development of the migraine headache. Consequently, my opinion that migraine is not a neurological disorder or brain disease.

Brain involvement means the initiation of the spreading excitation-depression phenomenon, usually in the part of the brain where vision is located. However, it can also happen in the area where sensation of the opposite side of the body resides or in the area that is involved in speech. It can progress forward from the vision part to the sensation part and, from there, to the speech part, resulting in visual symptoms, followed by sensory symptoms, and these, in turn, followed by difficulty speaking.

Fortunately for most people experiencing migraine aura, the spreading phenomenon dies out before it reaches the other areas of the brain. This also applies to those with so-called isolated migraine aura, in whom the migraine aura comes without headache.

We base the notion that there is a causal relation between the migraine aura and migraine headache mostly on the observation that one generally precedes the other. However, a relation in time, or temporal relation, is not the same as a cause-effect, or causal, relation, which is something we often forget.

The most important reason that aura symptoms, if present, appear before the onset of the headache may well be that as a tissue, the brain is much more reactive than the extracranial tissues, consisting of the muscles, tendons, blood vessels, nerves, and skin that make up our scalp.

Location

Concerning the migraine headache mechanism, I would like to address another issue here, and although coming at the end of the chapter, it is not any less important. It is the location in the head—the vascular compartment, so to say—where the vasodilation-inflammation mechanism of the migraine headache resides.

As discussed earlier, based on investigations conducted in migraineurs during and between migraine headaches, Professor Wolff concluded that the mechanism happens in the extracranial tissues—those on the outside of the skull—in particular in the frontotemporal area, which is between the forehead and the temple.

This is where the frontal branch of the superficial temporal artery is located, where we typically feel the pain of the migraine headache, and where cold or pressure often provides some relief. Applying pressure to the frontotemporal area, called Parry's compression test, in fact, we previously employed as an aid in the diagnosis of migraine.

As elaborately explained, in the first half of the last century, our understanding regarding the location of the migraine headache mechanism shifted from the brain to the tissues outside the skull, the extracranial tissues. We based this shift on solid experimental investigations conducted in humans and coming from two sides: disproving cerebral vasodilation as the vascular mechanism of the migraine headache and implicating extracranial vasodilation *and* inflammation.

Toward the end of the last century, another shift took place, moving the location of the migraine headache mechanism from extracranial to meningeal, or dural. This location brings us back into the skull but outside the brain, making it intracranial but extracerebral, implicating a structure called the pachymeninx, or dura mater.

The dura mater is a tendon-like membrane that covers the inside of the skull and is sensitive to pain in areas adjacent to the blood vessels. One of the major blood vessels in this membrane is the middle meningeal artery, which Professors Graham and Wolff observed to constrict only mildly in response to intravenous administration of the potent abortive migraine medication ergotamine.

As the meningeal, or dural, blood vessels lie inside the skull, increasing the cerebrospinal fluid, or CSF, pressure compresses them. This, in turn, mitigates their throbbing, which they found *not* to ameliorate migraine headaches, disproving their involvement as well.

Where did the shift that moved the location of the migraine headache mechanism from extracranial to meningeal, or dural, originate, and what was this shift based upon? Interestingly, it came from the same place where Professor Wolff started his migraine research in the 1920s, which was Massachusetts General Hospital, Harvard Medical School. We did not base it, however, on investigations conducted in migraineurs but on research performed in rodents, particularly rats and guinea pigs.

The focus of the research was the inflammatory component of neurogenic inflammation, mediated by the neuropeptide substance P; calcitonin gene-related peptide, or CGRP, is the peptide more involved in the vasodilatory component of the inflammation.

Stimulating the trigeminal ganglion was the technique employed to induce neurogenic inflammation in the heads of rats and guinea pigs. This is the ganglion, or nerve knot, from which the trigeminal nerve emerges that conveys sensory information, including pain, from the face and forehead, as well as from a large part of the dura mater, to the brain.

In those experiments, the abortive migraine medication ergotamine, which Professors Wolff and Graham also employed in their investigations, inhibited the inflammation in the dura mater but not in the extracranial tissues. Harvard scientists observed the same when they administered sumatriptan, an abortive migraine medication developed much later with a similar mode of action.

What led to the shift from extracranial to meningeal was that these abortive migraine medications did not block the neurogenic inflammation induced by trigeminal ganglion stimulation in the extracranial tissues but only in the dura mater. Therefore and importantly, we based this shift on research conducted in rodents and not in humans and, in addition, with an experimental approach that some have criticized as not physiological and, hence, not relevant to either species, rodent or human.

Chapter 8

How Do I Treat My Migraine Headaches?

Medications

Certainly, we do not treat migraine headaches with nonprescription medications, abortively or preventively. They are well beyond that! Instead, we should rely on prescription medications, preferably those specifically developed for the condition, which are the ones that are most likely to provide benefit. In addition, whatever we take, we need to make sure that we tolerate it well, without side effects; otherwise, it is not the right medication, and we should change it.

Over the almost fifty years that I have been treating migraine patients, I have pretty much tried everything to help them with their headaches and with their health in general. Regarding the latter, I cannot emphasize enough the importance of good physical and mental health for the long-term management of migraine.

Migraine does not exist in a vacuum, and consequently, we should not treat it as such, especially if long-term management is the goal which, as far as I am concerned, it should always be. Migraine is a chronic disorder in terms of the length of time people suffer from it, which is important to realize, also and maybe particularly in the context of treatment.

I will discuss the treatments that, over time, I have found effective and that I have stuck with. I may also mention those that I have specifically found not to be helpful, but will definitely focus on the ones that I have found beneficial for the majority of my patients. If I do not mention a particular treatment, it is probably because it did not work in my experience, or I did not find it particularly important to comment on.

Treatments need to be logical, make sense, and effectively address the issue, or issues, at hand. If a treatment is not effective, we should not continue it, especially if it involves taking a medication.

It should be clear that we only take medications that we tolerate well, without side effects, and that do what they are supposed to do. If this is not the case, we should discontinue them in dialogue with the physician or health care practitioner who prescribed them and under their guidance and direction. As it concerns prescription medications, the physician or health care practitioner is ultimately responsible, and we should respect that.

Abortive Treatment

By far the most important component of long-term migraine management is effective treatment of the individual headaches, referred to as acute or abortive treatment. I define effective treatment as one that provides *full* relief of headache within two hours. I italicized the word full because that is what we should aim for: total elimination of the headache, meaning a reduction of headache intensity to zero!

If you think that this is obvious, I can assure you from my experience that it is not. I always have to emphasize to patients that they should pursue the treatment of their headaches until they are fully gone. Once started, they should complete it unless they do not tolerate the medication well; if this is the case, it is not the right one, and we should change it.

I think that, on the one hand, many patients do not realize that they can obtain full relief of their headaches; on the other hand, they are generally content with a reduction to mild intensity, because that allows them to function again. Often, the diminution of nausea that comes with a reduction in headache intensity to mild permits them to resume normal functioning.

It is important, however, that we fully relieve migraine headaches abortively, because it makes no sense to suffer, especially if you do not have to. Maybe more significant, however, is that relieving migraine headaches fully decreases the likelihood of headache recurrence within twenty-four hours by two- to fourfold.

Headache recurrence is important because it not only prolongs the suffering but it also often requires taking more medication. The repeated intake of abortive migraine medications, especially vasoconstrictors and particularly those with caffeine, may lead to a vicious cycle that we know as rebound headache, from which it may be difficult to obtain relief.

Stomach

The biggest obstacle in the abortive treatment of migraine headaches is not the head, believe it or not, but the stomach. This is because we heavily rely on medications that we take by mouth, or orally, for whatever we treat, including migraine headaches.

The body does not take up, or absorb, medications in the stomach that we administer by mouth. They pass through the stomach and get absorbed in the small bowel, with some of them having preferential sites of absorption there. This, by the way, also applies to many nasal sprays with medications that are not working locally in the nose but aim for an effect in the body.

We put medications in nasal sprays for two reasons: either to treat the lining of the nose or for them to get absorbed into the body through it. Examples of the former are nasal sprays to treat nasal symptoms, such as congestion and postnasal drip from a head cold or allergies. Such sprays contain a decongestant, a corticosteroid, or an anti-allergy medication, the latter generally an antihistamine.

Related to migraine, the purpose of nasal sprays is to employ the lining of the nose to get the medication absorbed into the body. The lining of the nose is, however, not a very good surface for the absorption of medications—for example, in comparison to the rectum.

The other issue with nasal sprays is that we can only administer a small amount of fluid into the nose, which can only contain so much medication. People have been trying to get around this limitation by using powder nasal sprays; medications in powder form also stick better to the lining of the nose.

With liquid nasal sprays, which are the standard ones, fluid drips out of the nose in the front and in the back. The fluid that drips out in the front is lost, but we swallow what drips out in the back. The swallowed medication passes through the stomach and ends up in the small bowel, where it gets absorbed.

An additional issue with liquid nasal sprays is that most of the fluid stays in the lowest part of the nose, exposed to limited nasal lining, and drips out in the back. Therefore, it should not come as a surprise that of the sumatriptan liquid nasal spray for abortive migraine treatment, only approximately 15 percent is absorbed in the nose. For the liquid triptan nasal spray that contains zolmitriptan, this is a little better, but it is still only approximately 30 percent.

All of this means that the medications in those liquid triptan nasal sprays are mostly absorbed in the small bowel and, therefore, need to pass through the stomach. The situation is better with powder nasal sprays and those that also contain a so-called membrane permeability enhancer, which is a chemical that makes the lining of the nose absorb medications better.

Migraine headaches, due to the intense pain they generate, stimulate the sympathetic nervous system, and this has a pronounced effect on the stomach and on the large bowel. Nature created the sympathetic nervous system to prepare us for fight or flight under circumstances of threat. This would be a physical threat—that is, one hazardous to the integrity of the body—but mental threat or pain do very much the same.

Stress in general stimulates the sympathetic nervous system, allowing us to respond in a physical way, although that is mostly not relevant anymore, because the threat is mental, not physical. Allowing us to respond physically in the sense of fight or flight means shifting blood flow away from the stomach and the large bowel for the benefit of the muscles.

For the stomach and the large bowel, this also means not letting anything enter not to squander resources and expelling what is waste, the content of the large bowel. The latter results in a bowel movement, which can be with loose stool or diarrhea, as most of us probably know from personal experience when subjected to stress.

The closing down of the stomach results in cessation of the activity of the stomach that moves its content forward, called peristalsis, and in closure of the pyloric sphincter. This sphincter is the muscular ring that connects the stomach with the small bowel and that allows it to empty into the small bowel.

Once headache intensity escalates beyond a four on a ten-point scale, it progressively retards stomach emptying and closes the pyloric sphincter. This occurs regardless of nausea, although the more intense the headache, the worse the stomach retention and the higher the likelihood of nausea being present.

When the stomach retention is really bad, vomiting happens, and relief of the stomach distention resulting from the retention may temporarily ease the headache. We may also notice that when vomiting occurs, we throw up food that we ate a good time before and that is not digested because it never left the stomach.

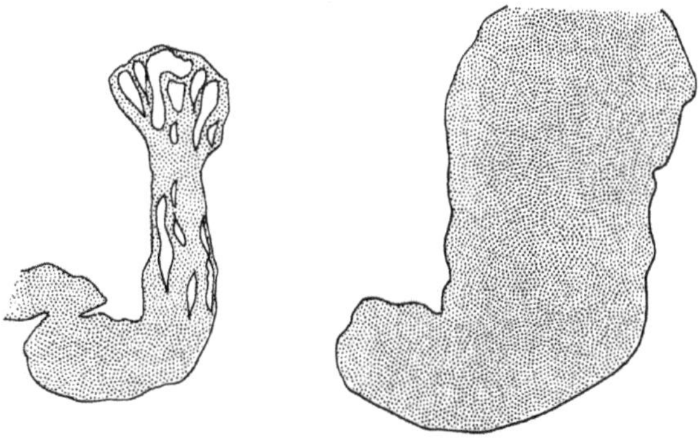

On the left, a normal stomach, actively contracting and moving its content forward through the pyloric sphincter into the small bowel; on the right, a stomach as it appears during a moderate or severe migraine headache, distended due to a lack of activity and filled with content that it cannot pass on to the small bowel because of the closed pyloric sphincter

It should be clear that the impact of the stimulated sympathetic nervous system on stomach emptying also has an effect on the efficacy of medications taken by mouth (or nasally). They are not absorbed as rapidly as they would otherwise, and speed of absorption strongly determines efficacy in abortive migraine treatment. This means that the faster the uptake of a medication into the body, the more powerful it is in relieving migraine headaches.

Headache Intensity

Studies with orally administered triptans have shown that if we take them at mild headache intensity, they provide full relief of headache within two hours in 80–85 percent. If we take them at moderate headache intensity, they provide full relief in 65 percent; whereas if we take them at severe intensity, this is the case in 45 percent only. All of this means that if you allow headache intensity to escalate to severe instead of treating at mild, you lose approximately half of the efficacy, literally down the drain or, in this case, down the gut.

Consequently, I strongly recommend against the use of nonprescription medications for the abortive treatment of migraine headaches. Taking them first, as some physicians and other health care practitioners unfortunately still advise, only allows time for the headache to progress, ultimately making the treatment much less effective.

Again, the goal of abortive migraine treatment is to fully relieve headaches within two hours, and nonprescription medications are just no match for these headaches. We should instead rely on migraine-specific medications, and when we administer them orally—or nasally, if we choose that route—we should take them at mild intensity for maximum benefit. I always emphasize to patients not to let headache intensity get beyond a four on a ten-point scale before initiating treatment and to use migraine-specific medications at all times.

Specific Medications

When it comes to specific migraine medications for abortive treatment, we have three classes: ergots, triptans, and gepants. The medications in all three classes predominantly work on the blood vessel, or vascular, component of the migraine headache mechanism. The ergots and triptans relieve migraine headaches by narrowing, or constricting, blood vessels, and the gepants block their widening specifically by calcitonin gene-related peptide, or CGRP.

In the context of migraine treatment, therefore, we can consider the ergots and triptans vasoconstrictors while the gepants are antivasodilators. The difference between them lies not so much in their efficacy in treating migraine headaches, which is approximately the same, but in the patients who should not use the vasoconstrictors because they are contraindicated.

Since vasoconstrictors narrow blood vessels, we should not use them in patients who already have issues with their blood vessels or who have high blood pressure that is not treated or not treated well. Issues with the blood vessels are important not only in relation to the heart and brain but in relation to the gut and legs as well.

The medical conditions that I am referring to are coronary artery disease with manifestations of angina or heart attack. From a brain perspective, the corresponding disorders are transient ischemic attack, or TIA, and stroke, the latter also referred to as brain attack. In the gut, such an attack would be ischemic colitis, manifesting itself with abdominal pain and rectal bleeding or bloody stool.

The underlying blood vessel condition is hardening of the arteries, or atherosclerosis, which limits the ability to walk longer distances if affecting the legs. Under all those circumstances, we should not use ergots or triptans, because as vasoconstrictors, they are contraindicated.

Ergotamine

The two ergots developed for abortive migraine treatment are ergotamine and dihydroergotamine, both out of the old box and marketed in 1921 and 1946 respectively. Dihydroergotamine is a derivative of ergotamine, synthesized to improve its tolerability. Across the board, ergots are quite toxic, however, and much more so than medications advanced since.

They are so toxic that they almost invariably cause nausea and sometimes vomiting as well, protracted at times. In addition and with frequent and prolonged exposure, they can also cause hallucinations, seizures, and gangrene, with fingers and toes dying off. We should not really prescribe them anymore, but they are still available, and patients still employ them.

We use ergotamine mostly in combination with caffeine to improve its absorption and potentiate its vasoconstrictor effect. It definitely needs the improvement of its absorption, because without it, it is rather poor at 5 percent or less. However, by itself, ergotamine is already a very potent vasoconstrictor, and a long-lasting one at that, keeping blood vessels narrowed for three to five days. This makes it an ideal medication for the treatment of severe migraine headaches that continue for days, such as we see with menstrual migraine headaches in particular.

The ergotamine-caffeine combination is available in tablet form and as a rectal suppository. However, it is not advisable to use the tablet because of very poor absorption, which is probably 1–2 percent only. It is a little better absorbed in the rectum with 5–6 percent of it taken up in the body.

The severe headaches that require a medication like ergotamine are almost invariably associated with nausea, if not with vomiting as well, making a tablet difficult to swallow and hold down anyway. Additionally, we should administer it with care not to aggravate the stomach complaints, especially if already present.

Therefore, I generally advise cutting the two-milligram ergotamine suppository in thirds and taking a third at a time every hour. If the suppository contains one milligram of the medication, along with caffeine dosed at one hundred milligrams, the patient should take half a suppository at a time. I recommend two milligrams as the maximum daily dose of ergotamine administered rectally with as much time as necessary to administer it as required for good tolerability.

Ergotamine is also available in a sublingual tablet—placed under the tongue and allowed to disintegrate in the mouth. It is doubtful whether any of it gets absorbed in the mouth, however, if only because it does not dissolve well in saliva.

The sublingual tablet contains two milligrams of the medication, and I used to prescribe it for abortive treatment in a disorder called cluster headache. This is a migraine-related condition that mostly affects men and presents with headaches that last one to two hours. They happen frequently, often daily and a couple of times per day, for weeks or months, referred to as clusters. In between the clusters, which we better call episodes, no headaches occur for months or sometimes years, referred to as remissions.

The abortive treatment of choice for cluster headache is with the sumatriptan injection, but we also use oxygen inhalation. Patients with cluster headache tolerate medications much better than those with migraine; ergotamine given in a single dose of two milligrams would make most migraineurs sick and cause them to vomit acutely. However, cluster headache patients tend to tolerate it well, as they also tolerate other medications well and without side effects.

Dihydroergotamine

In contrast to ergotamine, dihydroergotamine is available by itself only and in two formulations: nasal spray and injectable. As a vasoconstrictor, it is two times less potent than ergotamine; it is four times less toxic, causing nausea and vomiting. Consequently, patients tolerate it better, but it is still absorbed poorly unless, of course, given by injection.

The available liquid nasal spray contains 0.5 milligram of the medication per spray, and we administer one spray in each nostril, repeated after fifteen minutes. The total dose per treatment is two milligrams, of which, undoubtedly, most is not absorbed in the nose but in the small bowel.

The liquid nasal spray is also marketed with a special device that delivers the medication high up in the nasal cavity, from which it is supposedly absorbed better. With it, the patient administers the dose of 1.45 milligram as two sprays of 0.725 milligram, one in each nostril, which they can repeat once after an hour, if necessary.

In whatever way we administer the medication, the improvement is slow, because the ergots are slow-acting, and the benefit in terms of headache freedom is not well-established. The injectable dihydroergotamine is much more effective than the nasal spray, however, and I have used it extensively in the clinic for patients coming in with severe headache.

These patients usually seek treatment of severe headaches that they have struggled with for days without lasting relief. I treat them with dihydroergotamine in a dose of one milligram, administered subcutaneously, meaning under the skin, or intramuscularly, meaning in the muscle.

I always pretreat with an anti-nausea medication so as not to make their condition worse, even if the patient does not feel nauseated yet at the time of the visit. As an anti-nausea medication, I either use metoclopramide, ten milligrams intramuscularly, or ondansetron, four milligrams intramuscularly.

Under circumstances of prolonged severe headache, I prefer dihydroergotamine to sumatriptan because of its much longer duration of action. Sumatriptan is out of the body in approximately ten hours, and especially when given by injection, headache may return with a vengeance. This is generally not the case with dihydroergotamine, which stays in the body for at least five times longer, if not more.

The downside of using dihydroergotamine, however, is that it requires pretreatment with an anti-nausea medication, and in addition, benefit takes much longer to take effect. Sumatriptan administered by injection relieves severe headaches in twenty to forty minutes, while dihydroergotamine given by injection takes two to four hours to provide similar improvement.

We also administer dihydroergotamine intravenously as an infusion, often during hospitalization, to break what we call a migraine status, or status migrainosus. This refers to a migraine headache that has continued well beyond its usual duration, for which we often employ the arbitrary three-day mark. We base this on the erroneous assumption that migraine headaches last anywhere from four to seventy-two hours, which is nonsense.

Migraine Status

In general, migraine headaches minimally last a good part of the day, if not the whole day, requiring overnight sleep to be fully relieved, especially in adults. There is no maximum duration, and I personally consider it a migraine status if the headache, as aforementioned, continues well beyond its usual duration for the particular patient, whatever that is.

An effective treatment for status migrainosus is the administration of dihydroergotamine by injection. However, to receive such treatment, the patient needs to travel to the clinic, which can be difficult, especially if there is nausea and vomiting. An alternative is to prescribe a dose or two of a fast- and short-acting sleeping medication, or hypnotic, like zolpidem, to put the patient to sleep for the night.

If the headache has been present severely for days, this will not be adequate, however, and we have to resort to a three-day course of a corticosteroid. Under such circumstances, I prescribe prednisone in a dose of fifteen milligrams four times per day for one day, ten milligrams four times per day for one day, and five milligrams four times per day for one day. I always advise patients to take the medication with meals and at bedtime with some food as well to protect the stomach.

If the headache is associated with significant tightness of the neck, shoulder, and upper back muscles, which is often the case, I add diazepam to relax them. Without the muscle relaxant, the headache may flare up again after the prednisone course is finished, which defeats the purpose. I prefer to prescribe it four times per day as well in a dose of one to five milligrams, depending on the patient's tolerance.

It is extremely important that the patient discontinues all medications taken abortively for headache, including nonprescription medications. The prednisone, with or without diazepam, should be allowed to do the job of relieving the migraine headache by itself, which it will generally do in twelve to twenty-four hours.

Rebound Headache

If we employ an ergot for abortive migraine treatment, which currently should be rarely, if at all, it should not be used more than once per week on average because of its long duration of action which, as aforementioned, is three to five days. We want to prevent it from building up in the body, which happens upon repeat administration within its duration of action.

The effect of the medication wearing off leads to rebound headache, nowadays called medication overuse headache, a vicious cycle in which a new headache develops every time the effect of the abortive medication wears off. In this way, we bring about a situation where the medication becomes less and less effective, probably because the headaches are getting worse and worse.

In addition, it produces a decrease or loss of response to preventive treatment, although this may be less an issue with the newer and more potent preventive migraine medications, such as the calcitonin gene-related peptide, or CGRP, antibodies and gepants.

To illustrate the above point, I saw a man who experienced migraine headaches approximately every five days, which he treated with a dihydroergotamine injection. As migraine headaches rarely, if ever, occur with that kind of regularity, I suspected rebound headache and advised him to discontinue the medication.

In order to help him through the withdrawal headache, I prescribed the aforementioned prednisone course, but for six days rather than three days because of dihydroergotamine's long duration of action. After he was done with the course and to my great surprise, he appeared to have cluster headache, which I treated successfully with appropriate medications.

Triptans

The triptans are the successors of the ergots, and we based their development on an animal migraine model validated with the ergots, which I did as a PhD student in experimental pharmacology. Consequently, the triptans have a similar, if not the same, mode of action in migraine, but they are different in several ways that make them more effective, better tolerated, and safer.

Like the ergots, they are vasoconstrictors and, hence, they have the same contraindications. In terms of their molecular size, they are much smaller than the ergots which are, in fact, small proteins. Consequently, the body absorbs them better and breaks them down more easily, resulting in a faster onset and shorter duration of action.

Administered orally at mild headache intensity, the triptans fully relieve migraine headaches within two hours in 80–85 percent, which is approximately 65 percent when taken at moderate intensity. Administered intranasally, they are slightly more effective; given subcutaneously, they relieve severe migraine headaches in twenty to forty minutes.

With the exception of the injection, the triptans generally provide benefit for at least twenty-four hours, assuming that the headache is *fully* relieved. If not, it recurs within twenty-four hours in one-quarter to one-third of headaches treated. We can improve this, however, by two- to fourfold if we pursue the treatment to the extent of full headache relief, as opposed to leaving residual headache behind even if mild in intensity.

Patients generally tolerate the triptans well with minimal, if any, side effects. The most common side effects are tingling in the fingers and tightness of the throat. Nasal congestion, postnasal drip, and a foul taste in the mouth or in the back of the throat are side effects of nasal sprays in general, regardless of the medication they contain.

The six-milligram sumatriptan injection generally has side effects that come on rather quickly which, in combination with their intensity, can be such that they cause a panic attack. They consist of a hot feeling that ascends the body like a hot flash, associated with a feeling of tightness in the upper chest, throat, back of the neck, and head. These side effects develop within five to ten minutes and last the same duration, after which the headache is rapidly relieved.

The sumatriptan injection also comes in dosages of three milligrams and four milligrams, which patients generally tolerate better while similarly effective. I prefer those, which I have patients repeat after an hour if the headache is not fully relieved.

If repeat dosing is generally required and they tolerate the medication well, I increase the dose to six milligrams. If the headache is mostly gone but not completely, alternatively, the patient can follow up with a sumatriptan tablet to relieve it fully.

Combining the sumatriptan injection with the tablet has the additional benefit of securing headache freedom for at least twenty-four hours. With use of the injection alone, headache commonly returns after twelve to sixteen hours, and it may do so with such vengeance that another injection is required.

The maximum daily dose of sumatriptan administered by injection is twelve milligrams, which amounts to two six-milligram injections, three four-milligram injections, or four three-milligram injections.

When the initial treatment is not with the sumatriptan injection but with a triptan tablet or nasal spray, it is prudent to wait two hours to determine the benefit, because it takes longer for the medication to get absorbed. If the headache is not fully relieved at that point and tolerability is good, it should be repeated immediately to obtain the cumulative benefit.

Patients should always use the optimum dose of the triptan, and if repeat dosing is necessary more often than not and tolerability is good, they should take double the optimum dose at the onset. Three of the triptans—eletripan, sumatriptan, and zolmitriptan—are available in double-the-optimum-dose tablets. Therefore, I like to prescribe them, because they can be broken into halves to obtain the optimum doses, and progression to double the optimum dose is easy.

Seven

In total, there are seven triptans on the market, and all of them have a maximum daily dose that is important to keep in mind. If repeat dosing is necessary, which patients should do only if tolerability is good, they should always do so with intervals no longer than two hours to obtain the cumulative benefit.

The following table lists the seven oral triptans in alphabetical order, along with their tablet strengths, optimum doses, and maximum daily doses.

Table: Oral triptans with their tablet strengths, optimum doses, and maximum daily doses

Triptan Name	Tablet Strengths	Optimum Doses	Maximum Daily Doses
Almotriptan	6.25 and 12.5 milligrams	12.5 milligrams	25 milligrams
Eletriptan	20 and 40 milligrams	20 milligrams	80 milligrams
Frovatriptan	2.5 milligrams	2.5 milligrams	7.5 milligrams
Naratriptan	1 and 2.5 milligrams	2.5 milligrams	5 milligrams
Rizatriptan	5 and 10 milligrams	10 milligrams*	30 milligrams*
Sumatriptan	25, 50, and 100 milligrams	50 milligrams	200 milligrams
Zolmitriptan	2.5 and 5 milligrams	2.5 milligrams	10 milligrams

*With simultaneous use of propranolol, the optimum dose of rizatriptan is five milligrams, and its maximum daily dose is fifteen milligrams.

As mentioned, only eletriptan, sumatriptan, and zolmitriptan are available in tablet strengths that represent double the optimum dose. These are indicated if the patient generally needs to repeat the optimum dose to obtain full headache relief and tolerates the medication well without side effects. If the headache is not fully relieved, the oral triptan should be repeated after two hours with the exception of naratriptan, which the patient should repeat after four hours, because it takes longer to get absorbed.

Four of the oral triptans come in tablet strengths that we should not employ except under certain circumstances. This is the case for rizatriptan, of which we should prescribe the five-milligram tablet exclusively in patients on propranolol. This particular beta-blocker inhibits the breakdown of the medication by the liver, which is the reason for using half the optimum dose and for the lower maximum daily dose of fifteen milligrams.

For almotriptan, naratriptan, and sumatriptan, the lowest tablet strengths are on the market only because they represent the lowest effective dosages. Sometimes, they are mistaken for pediatric doses, but those do not exist for the triptans; in teenagers and adolescents, we should use the listed optimum doses.

For two triptans—rizatriptan and zolmitriptan—orally disintegrating tablets are available as well, which we refer to as ODT. The patient places these on or under the tongue allowing them to disintegrate in the mouth. The medication dissolves in the saliva, which the patient swallows down for it to get absorbed in the small bowel.

The common perception is that medications taken this way work faster, but the opposite is generally true, because it takes time for the saliva to travel down to the stomach. Therefore, I recommend that when the prescription calls for an orally disintegrating tablet, the patient swallows it down like a regular tablet.

We often also consider that orally disintegrating tablets are easier to use because patients can take them without water. However, the triptan tablets are generally small enough to be swallowed down without water as well.

We may also think about them as ideal when nausea is present, but if this is the case, the headache is at least moderately severe, if not severe. It is then of an intensity that it has already stimulated the sympathetic nervous system to the extent of slowing stomach emptying, thereby affecting the absorption and, hence, the efficacy of the medication.

Nasal Sprays

Two of the triptans—sumatriptan and zolmitriptan—are also available as liquid nasal sprays. The sumatriptan spray comes in two dosages—five milligrams and twenty milligrams—while the zolmitriptan spray comes in the dose of five milligrams only.

When the sumatriptan nasal spray is used, we should prescribe the twenty-milligram dose, which the patient can repeat once after two hours, if necessary, with a maximum daily dose of forty milligrams. When the zolmitriptan nasal spray is used, they can repeat it as well after two hours, if necessary, with a maximum daily dose of ten milligrams.

The liquid nasal sprays are only slightly more effective than the oral tablets, because not more than 15 percent of intranasally administered sumatriptan and 30 percent of intranasally administered zolmitriptan is absorbed in the nose. Consequently, most intranasally administered medication—that is, 85 percent of sumatriptan and 70 percent of zolmitriptan—is absorbed in the small bowel as if taken by mouth.

This may be better with the sumatriptan powder nasal spray, for which the dose is twenty-two milligrams (two times eleven milligrams), which the patient can repeat once after two hours, if necessary, with a maximum daily dose of forty-four milligrams.

This particular nasal spray comes with a special device; the patient puts one side in the mouth and the other in the nose and then blows the powder into the nose. The act of blowing makes the soft palate close off the passage from the nose to the throat, keeping the medication in the nasal cavity for enhanced absorption.

The nasal absorption may also be better with the sumatriptan liquid nasal spray that contains a so-called membrane permeability enhancer. The dose of this spray is ten milligrams, which the patient can repeat every hour, if necessary, with a maximum daily dose of three sprays, or thirty milligrams.

In Europe, sumatriptan comes as a rectal suppository as well in dosages of 12.5 milligrams and 25 milligrams. The recommended dose is 25 milligrams, which the patient can repeat, if necessary, after two hours with a maximum of 50 milligrams per day.

Gepants

The gepants are the newest kids on the block when it comes to abortive migraine medications. In opposition to the ergots and triptans, which are vasoconstrictors, the gepants are antivasodilators and, hence, do not have the contraindications of uncontrolled high blood pressure, or hypertension, and conditions affecting the blood vessels of the heart, brain, gut, or legs.

The gepants are contraindicated, however, with the simultaneous use of medications that strongly inhibit a liver enzyme system known as CYP3A4. This enzyme system is important for the breakdown of the gepants, and when strongly inhibited, it causes more to remain in the body and for longer. This, in turn, may bring about more, or more pronounced side effects, which for the gepants in general are drowsiness, fatigue, nausea, and constipation.

The medications that we know best to strongly inhibit the CYP3A4 liver enzyme system are those used for the treatment of viral or fungal infections, but others do so as well. The simultaneous use of a strong CYP3A4 inhibitor is also a contraindication for the aforementioned abortive migraine medications—dihydroergotamine, almotriptan, and eletriptan.

The gepants are antivasodilators in the sense that they block the blood vessel widening, or vasodilatory, effect of calcitonin gene-related peptide, or CGRP. In order to induce vasodilation, calcitonin gene-related peptide needs to bind to and stimulate its receptors on the blood vessels, and the gepants block access to those receptors.

Therefore, we refer to them as small molecule CGRP receptor antagonists, with an antagonist being a medication that attaches itself to a receptor but does not stimulate it. A medication that binds to a receptor and stimulates it, on the other hand, we call an agonist.

Examples of agonist medications are the ergots and triptans reviewed earlier, which relieve migraine headaches by attaching themselves to and stimulating the so-called serotonin 1B receptors on blood vessels. These receptors are predominantly located on the blood vessels in the head, which dilate and become inflamed as part of the migraine headache mechanism.

The ergots in particular stimulate numerous other receptors as well, such as the serotonin 2A receptors on the blood vessels in the heart and the alpha-adrenergic receptors on the blood vessels in the legs. Through stimulation of dopamine receptors in the brain stem, they cause the nausea and vomiting for which they are so notorious.

Three

The three gepants that are available for the abortive treatment of migraine are rimegepant, ubrogepant, and zavegepant. They are very similar to each other in terms of efficacy, tolerability, and safety.

Their efficacy is similar to that of the triptans, but their duration of action is longer, which means that they provide somewhat longer-lasting benefit. In general, patients tolerate the gepants as well as they do the oral triptans; if side effects occur, they tend to be drowsiness or fatigue with the gepants and tingling or muscle tightness with the triptans.

Rimegepant is available in one tablet strength only, which is seventy-five milligrams, while ubrogepant comes in tablets of fifty milligrams and one hundred milligrams. The rimegepant tablet is an orally disintegrating tablet, or ODT, which the patient can swallow down or place on or under the tongue, allowing it to disintegrate in the mouth.

The medication subsequently dissolves in the saliva, which the patient swallows down for it to get absorbed in the small bowel. Ubrogepant, on the other hand, is available in a regular tablet only that the patient swallows down; zavegepant comes in a liquid spray for nasal administration.

The patient cannot repeat the seventy-five-milligram rimegepant tablet within twenty-four hours while they can repeat the ubrogepant every two hours, if necessary, with a maximum daily dose of two hundred milligrams. The zavegepant nasal spray comes in a strength of ten milligrams, which like rimegepant can be administered only once in twenty-four hours.

The only true medical indication for the use of gepants as abortive migraine medications is the presence of triptan contraindications. These are, as mentioned, conditions affecting the blood vessels of the heart, brain, gut, or legs or high blood pressure that is not treated or not treated well.

Inflammation

Along with vasodilation, inflammation is part of the migraine headache mechanism as well and probably of at least equal importance. We can address it with anti-inflammatory medications, such as the aforementioned prednisone prescribed for the treatment of migraine status, or status migrainosus.

It is a corticosteroid—or steroid, for short—a potent medication that we should employ sparingly because of potentially serious side effects. For the abortive treatment of migraine, we need to give it in a relatively high dose, such as sixty milligrams, and it easily takes twelve to twenty-four hours to provide benefit.

However, there is also another group of anti-inflammatory medications, referred to as nonsteroidal anti-inflammatory drugs, or NSAIDs. As the name implies, they are not corticosteroids or steroids; hence, they do not have the limitations in frequency of use that those have.

In addition to decreasing inflammation, the nonsteroidal anti-inflammatory drugs provide pain relief, because they are pain medications, or analgesics. The best-known member of this class is aspirin, and therefore, we also refer to them as aspirin-like analgesics. Other well-known members are ibuprofen and naproxen sodium which, like aspirin, are available as nonprescription medications.

As pain medications, they are not specific to migraine, because they relieve pain in general. However, they also treat inflammation, as their name implies, which makes them, at least in part, specific to migraine.

As they are only partially specific, they generally do not relieve migraine headaches as effectively as the migraine-specific abortive medications—that is, ergots, triptans, and gepants. This means that if we employ them for migraine abortion, we have to administer relatively high doses, such as 1,000 milligrams of aspirin, 800 milligrams of ibuprofen, or 880 milligrams of naproxen sodium.

However, even taking such high dosages may not be sufficient for good efficacy, and we may also need to enhance their absorption. We can do so in several ways, and I have extensive experience pretreating with medications that stimulate stomach emptying, in particular metoclopramide.

Prior to the advent of the triptans in the early nineties, I often recommended taking ten milligrams of the medication for migraine abortion, followed in fifteen minutes by one thousand milligrams of soluble aspirin. This kind of aspirin dissolves in water, which makes it easier on the stomach and, at the same time, gets it ready for absorption in the small bowel.

Metoclopramide is an anti-nausea medication that uniquely stimulates the stomach to empty out faster into the small bowel. The combination of a relatively high dose of aspirin, its dissolved status, and stimulation of stomach emptying makes this approach reasonably effective for migraine abortion. Instead of metoclopramide, we can also use a medication called domperidone in the same dose of ten milligrams.

The difference between the two is that domperidone, unlike metoclopramide, does not enter the brain. As a result, it does not have the potential side effect of restlessness, called akathisia, that the latter has, although it rarely occurs when taken by mouth.

Akathisia is a common side effect, however, when we administer metoclopramide intravenously, and therefore, I do not recommend that we give it this way. For the same reason, other physicians combine it with diphenhydramine whenever they administer it intravenously to prevent this annoying side effect.

We treat the restlessness, or akathisia, whenever it happens and for whatever reason, with diphenhydramine, which is an antihistamine that, as such, causes drowsiness. I do not like to give it in the context of treating migraine headaches abortively, because I like the patient to be able to return to normal functioning. Administering them a potentially sedating medication like diphenhydramine, which almost invariably causes drowsiness, obviously gets us further away from this goal.

Another way of making an aspirin-like analgesic more effective for abortive migraine treatment is combining it with caffeine. A relatively high dose of the aspirin-like analgesic is still required, but the added caffeine, usually in a dose of fifty milligrams or one hundred milligrams, improves its absorption. It has the additional benefit of being a vasoconstrictor, thus tightening the widened blood vessels in the head that contribute to the migraine headache.

Multiple combinations of aspirin-like analgesics and caffeine are available as nonprescription headache or migraine medications. However, I generally do not recommend them for migraine abortion for two reasons. First, specific migraine medications usually provide better, if not much better, benefit. Second, their frequent intake gives rise to two treatment complications I regularly encounter in medical practice: rebound headache and a toxic effect on the stomach.

Treatment Complications

Rebound headache, nowadays also called medication overuse headache, stems from the regular use of vasoconstrictors—medications that narrow blood vessels—for headache, including migraine. When we take such a vasoconstrictor medication frequently enough to accumulate in the body, headache ensues every time its effect wears off. Rebound vasodilation is the cause of those headaches, and even non-migraineurs may be familiar with it in the setting of coffee withdrawal.

People generally do not realize that caffeine is not only a potent vasoconstrictor, but also that its effect in the body lasts as long as two to three days. This means that if we take a caffeine-containing medication for headache even as infrequently as every other day, the caffeine builds up in the body and potentially causes rebound headache. Therefore, I recommend that those medications, whether prescription or nonprescription, not be used for headache more than twice per week on average.

Patients should not take an ergot medication for headache more than once per week, because its vasoconstrictor effect lasts twice as long as that of caffeine. On the other hand, they can take a triptan daily but not more than once per day due to their duration of action generally being less than a day.

The gepants do not have this particular rebound problem, because they are not vasoconstrictors, and nonsteroidal anti-inflammatory pain medications without caffeine do not have this limitation in frequency of use either. They do not cause rebound headache.

We know that both steroidal and nonsteroidal anti-inflammatory medications with frequent or prolonged use are harmful to the stomach. They weaken the protective layer that lines the stomach, allowing the acid made by the stomach to irritate its wall and cause inflammation, known as gastritis.

Caffeine-containing, aspirin-like medications are the worst in this regard, because caffeine stimulates the stomach to produce more acid, creating a situation of more acid and less protection against its potentially harmful impact.

Stomach inflammation, or gastritis, comes with tiny ulcerations, through which we lose blood in a way that is not visible, known as occult blood loss. It may not amount to more than a drop or a couple of drops per day, but it adds up over time and, over the course of years, leads to iron deficiency and anemia.

Both conditions contribute to fatigue, which is a common cause of headaches, including migraine headaches. Therefore, if we use a nonsteroidal anti-inflammatory medication for the abortive treatment of migraine headaches, I prefer the ones that do not contain caffeine.

We developed two such medications—diclofenac and celecoxib—in specific formulations for abortive migraine treatment. Diclofenac is available as a powder that dissolves in water and contains fifty milligrams of the medication. However, patients can take it only once in twenty-four hours for migraine abortion.

Celecoxib comes in an oral solution that contains 120 milligrams of the medication, in addition to a solubility enhancer to improve its absorption. Like the diclofenac formulation, patients can also take it only once in twenty-four hours. This means that they cannot repeat either one within twenty-four hours and that a single dose has to do the job, relieving migraine headaches fully within two hours.

Of course, we can also take those two nonsteroidal anti-inflammatory medications after pretreatment with metoclopramide or domperidone to improve their absorption further and, consequently, their efficacy.

As patients cannot repeat either medication within twenty-four hours, it is important that the one dose fully relieves the migraine headaches, with or without pretreatment. If not, there is a reasonable chance that the headache builds up again later in the day, requiring the patient to take another medication, which is far from ideal and something we should avoid.

Headache Development

Knowledge of how the migraine headaches develop in a given patient is essential for securing effective abortive treatment, again defined as treatment that *fully* relieves them within two hours. If a physician or other health care practitioner does not inquire about this particular aspect of the headaches, securing effective abortive treatment is an illusion.

First, it is important to know whether the migraine headaches are generally present on awakening in the morning, come on during the day, or wake the patient from sleep at night. Starting with the latter, only severe headaches are intense enough to disrupt sleep and, hence, wake the patient. In that case, no further questioning is required, and we have to assume that stomach emptying is impaired at the time of treatment, even without the presence of nausea.

Generally, the most effective treatment of headaches that wake the patient from sleep at night is the sumatriptan injection, which I prefer to start at the three-milligram or four-milligram dose because of better tolerability. If the headache is still moderate or severe after an hour, I recommend that they repeat it once. If this does the job and the patient tolerates the medication well, I increase the dose to six milligrams.

Patients generally do not tolerate the six-milligram dose of sumatriptan as well as the three-milligram or four-milligram dose. Although the side effects of the six-milligram dose can be intense, their duration is relatively short, lasting five to ten minutes at the most.

If the medication has significantly diminished the headache after an hour but it is not gone yet, the patient should take a fifty-milligram sumatriptan tablet at that point to relieve it fully. They can repeat the tablet, if necessary, after two hours, and all of it constitutes one intake, although spread out over several hours.

If the migraine headaches are present on awakening in the morning, it is important to know what their intensity usually is at that time. For this purpose, I like the patient to rate it on a ten-point scale with ten being the worst pain possible.

If the headache is mild—that is, up to a three or four on the ten-point scale—the patient should initiate treatment immediately and without hesitation, preferably with a migraine-specific medication in oral formulation, such as a triptan or a gepant.

As to the triptan, I prefer sumatriptan, because it has been on the market the longest, since 1991, thus well over thirty years. Consequently, we have extensive experience with it, also in specific patient populations, such as teenagers or adolescents and pregnant women.

It is readily available and cheap, certainly in its tablet formulation, which costs approximately one United States dollar per tablet regardless of the strength. Finally, it comes in an injectable formulation as well with an auto-injector for easy self-administration. This is a wonderful product to have handy if the headache gets out of control and out of reach of orally administered medication.

For the sumatriptan tablet, fifty milligrams is the optimum dose, which I always recommend that patients repeat after two hours if the headache is not *fully* relieved and the tolerability is good, which it generally is. If repeat dosing is usually required to obtain full headache relief and they tolerate the medication well, I switch to the one-hundred-milligram dose. If necessary, they can also repeat this after two hours because its maximum daily dose is two hundred milligrams.

If the headache on awakening in the morning is moderate in intensity, I use the one-hundred-milligram sumatriptan tablet to see whether, with the higher dose, I can overcome the delayed emptying of the stomach that is present at that intensity.

If the headache on awakening is severe, I recommend the use of the sumatriptan injection, starting with the three-milligram or four-milligram dose and, if necessary, increasing it to six milligrams.

The regular liquid nasal spray of the medication is not potent enough for severe headaches, because its efficacy is not much better than that of the tablet. The powder nasal spray and the one with the membrane permeability enhancer may be sufficiently effective here, however.

They may be beneficial when the one-hundred-milligram tablet—if necessary, repeated after two hours—does not do the job for moderate headaches. Again, full relief of headache is the goal of treatment, if possible accomplished within two hours and without side effects.

If the migraine headaches come on during the day, which is fortunately most often the case, it is important to know how long they generally take to build to their maximum intensity. Usually, migraine headaches escalate over one to two hours—rarely longer but sometimes shorter. This should allow plenty of time to initiate treatment at mild intensity, which means up to a three or four on the ten-point scale.

We can initiate treatment as aforementioned, for example, with the fifty-milligram sumatriptan tablet—if necessary, repeated after two hours. If the patient does not tolerate the medication well, I will switch to another triptan and determine my choice based on the nature of the side effects and on the observed benefit.

Side Effects

It is important to distinguish between specific and nonspecific side effects of medications. The nonspecific side effect is fatigue, which I think is the body's response to anything put into it that does not belong there.

Here, it is important to remember that medications are toxins. The Latin word for *medication* is *pharmacon*, which means both "remedy" and "poison." Nowadays, we also have biologics as medications, such as antibodies, to which this may not apply because they are either human or humanized—that is, mostly human.

Fatigue is especially prone to happen as a medication's side effect if low energy is already a problem for the patient. It lowers their tolerance in general, under which circumstance fatigue is more likely to occur. Changing to another medication may help, but it is generally more effective to identify the cause or causes of the low energy and treat them. Doing so is also an important step in the overall management of headaches, including migraine, especially when they happen frequently.

A common, specific side effect of sumatriptan is nausea, usually mild in intensity and nothing compared to that often encountered with the ergot medications ergotamine and dihydroergotamine. The origin of the nausea is also different in the sense that the ergots cause it by stimulating dopamine receptors in the brain stem while sumatriptan can cause it because it slightly retards stomach emptying.

I have not found nausea to be an issue with the other triptans, such as rizatriptan or zolmitriptan. These two are as effective as sumatriptan in relieving migraine headaches, with rizatriptan working slightly faster but also somewhat shorter. In practice, I prefer zolmitriptan to rizatriptan, however, mostly because, like sumatriptan, it comes in a tablet strength that is double the optimum dose, making working with it easier and cheaper. Consequently, I am inclined to prescribe it as the second triptan, with rizatriptan third.

Eletriptan falls in the same category as rizatriptan, sumatriptan, and zolmitriptan in terms of its efficacy in relieving migraine headaches. However, the simultaneous use of a strong CYP3A4 inhibitor, such as an antifungal or antiviral medication, is a contraindication for its use. The same is true for almotriptan, which may be a little less effective in relieving migraine headaches, but patients tend to tolerate it better, if that is an issue.

Generally the best-tolerated triptans, however, are frovatriptan and naratriptan, especially when it comes to the typical triptan side effects, such as tingling in the fingers or tightness of the throat. In clinical trials, these triptans show lower efficacy than the others, but this is not necessarily the case in an individual patient. For example, I have seen naratriptan work effectively in patients when a medication like sumatriptan fails them.

It is very important to find an abortive migraine medication that the patient tolerates well, because when taken orally and for maximum benefit, they need to take it at mild headache intensity. Patients are reluctant to do so when they experience side effects, especially when their ability to function is impaired by fatigue or drowsiness.

The latter are specific side effects of the gepants, but they only happen in a low and single-digit percent of patients. The same is true for the nausea and constipation occasionally seen with them. Like for almotriptan and eletriptan, the simultaneous use of a strong CYP3A4 inhibitor, such as an antifungal or antiviral medication, is a contraindication to their use.

Patients can repeat any triptan in its optimum dose after two hours and should do so if the tolerability is good and the headache is not *fully* relieved. Of the three gepants available for migraine abortion, they can only repeat ubrogepant after two hours, if necessary, with a maximum of two hundred milligrams per day. This makes it imperative that, with the use of either rimegepant or zavegepant, they fully relieve the headaches, because the patient cannot repeat them within twenty-four hours.

Patients can combine gepants and triptans, but it makes it more complicated if they require two medications to relieve their migraine headaches fully. Simplicity is key, and this is the case with everything, including the abortive treatment of migraine.

An interesting observation is that the lower the intensity of the headache when taking a medication, the better patients tolerate it even though more of it gets absorbed. The increased absorption translates into better efficacy, and I think that the close-to-normal condition of the body at lower headache intensity conveys better tolerability.

Migraine headaches affect the body as a whole, and the impact accelerates with increasing headache intensity, quickly lowering its tolerance to anything put into it, including medications.

Combining Medications

If the patient tolerates the triptan well, takes it in the appropriate dose for the headache intensity treated, and repeats it after two hours but the migraine headaches are nevertheless not yet fully relieved, they should take it along with a nonsteroidal anti-inflammatory medication.

For this purpose, a combination product is available that contains eighty-five milligrams of sumatriptan and five hundred milligrams of naproxen sodium, which the patient can repeat once after two hours, if necessary, with a maximum of two tablets per day.

Of course, it is not necessary to use this particular combination product, and the patient can just as easily take any triptan tablet together with 500 milligrams of aspirin, 400 milligrams of ibuprofen, or 440 milligrams of naproxen sodium. We can do the same, if necessary, with a gepant.

We can proceed similarly if the triptan or gepant does fully relieve the migraine headaches, but there is residual sensitivity of the scalp, which is what we can see, especially with headaches that continue for days. In this case, lingering inflammation of the scalp renders it tender to the touch and makes combing one's hair uncomfortable.

We often allude to this scalp tenderness as allodynia, but that is not exactly the correct term, because allodynia refers to pain from an ordinarily painless stimulus. What we are dealing with here is sensitivity of the scalp due to residual inflammation while allodynia is due to nerve damage, which is not the case with migraine headaches.

Lasmiditan

A specific abortive migraine medication that I have not mentioned yet is lasmiditan, which is unfortunately one with a number of problems. In terms of relieving migraine headaches, it is similarly effective as the triptans and the gepants, but patients do not to tolerate it well. Light-headedness or dizziness is a frequent side effect, but fatigue and drowsiness are common as well.

For an oral medication that the patient needs to take when headache intensity is mild, these side effects are obviously a deterrent. They are also the reason that patients should not drive or operate machinery for at least eight hours after using it. The dose is fifty milligrams, one hundred milligrams, or two hundred milligrams, which the patient can take only once in twenty-four hours and, therefore, must provide *full* headache relief to be satisfactory.

Like the gepants, lasmiditan is not a vasoconstrictor; consequently, we can employ it in patients with contraindications to the ergots and triptans due to conditions affecting the blood vessels of the heart, brain, gut, or legs or high blood pressure that is not treated or not treated well.

The medication has a unique mode of action in treating migraine headaches; by stimulating so-called serotonin 1F receptors, it inhibits the release of the chemicals from the pain nerve fibers that cause neurogenic inflammation. Unlike any of the other specific abortive migraine medications mentioned, it enters the brain and, therefore, potentially blocks the transmission of pain signals in the central nervous system as well, a distinct property of the medication.

The very fact, however, that it enters the brain unfortunately also accounts for the aforementioned tolerability issues. If the brain does not have to be within your therapeutic target, it is better to leave it out of it, especially from a tolerability perspective.

This is definitely the case with migraine treatment, whether abortive or preventive, which we have shown to be effective, if not very effective, with medications that do not enter the brain. Hence, influencing the brain is not required to effectively abort or prevent migraine headaches, and much of the progress we have made in terms of tolerability relates to this particular issue.

Chapter 9

What Can I Do to Prevent Those Headaches?

Headache Triggers

We can prevent migraine headaches in three ways: first, by identifying what triggers them and by avoiding those triggers; second, by improving our general health, mental and physical; and third, by taking an effective and well-tolerated preventive migraine medication, preferably one specifically developed for this purpose.

The list of headache triggers is long, and in addition, I have come to understand that there are no migraine triggers, only headache triggers. Whether they cause headache or migraine depends on the individual, with migraine being a genetically determined and inherited vulnerability to intense headaches.

In general, headaches do not develop without a reason; they do not just fall out of a clear blue sky. Something brings them on, although it may not always be clear what. I hear it from patients both ways: either nothing brings them on, or everything does.

For me, these two statements essentially mean the same and ask for a systematic approach—first, identifying the triggers and then avoiding them wherever possible. As several triggers working together generally bring on headache, as opposed to a single trigger acting alone, it is often more an issue of preventing triggers from compounding than avoiding them.

Menstrual Cycle

By far the most potent trigger of headaches, including migraine headaches, is the menstrual cycle. In order to identify it as a trigger, the patient needs to keep a diary of the headaches, on the one hand, and of the days of menstruation, on the other. As it is such an important trigger, I recommend that all menstruating women keep such a diary until it is clear whether the headaches happen in relation to the menstrual cycle and if so, when.

There are three times in the menstrual cycle that women are most vulnerable to headaches and, consequently, to migraine headaches. The first and most important one is one or two days before menstruation, when the biggest drop in blood estrogen level occurs. The second one is midcycle, at the time of ovulation, when the blood estrogen level also falls but to a lesser extent. The third one is at the tail end of menstruation due to the blood estrogen level, low during menstruation, rising again.

The situation is a little different with women on cyclical estrogen-containing birth control. Then the migraine headaches happen along with the vaginal bleeding in the week off due to hormone withdrawal.

Estrogen-containing birth control suppresses ovulation and, therefore, the vaginal bleeding associated with its cyclical use, we should not call menstruation. We define the latter as the shedding of the lining of the womb, or uterus, due to the hormonal changes brought about by ovulation. With estrogen-containing birth control, there is no ovulation, and the vaginal bleeding is due to withdrawal from its progestin component.

The estrogen withdrawal that accompanies it causes the headache, usually four days after the interruption of the birth control. Women generally start the estrogen-containing birth control on a Sunday and then take it for three weeks with the bleeding and headache occurring on the Wednesday of the fourth week, which is the week off or the placebo week.

Migraineurs in general should not use estrogen-containing birth control, because it is likely to make their headaches worse. This is especially the case when on it, the headaches happen consistently during the week off or during the placebo week, as just described, indicating that they are hormonally sensitive.

It is good to know whether the headaches occur in relation to the menstrual cycle and, if so, when exactly they are most likely to happen. This, if anything, allows the woman to be prepared, both in terms of treatment and in terms of avoiding additional triggers that may make the situation worse.

Migraine headaches that occur premenstrually—one or two days before menstruation—tend to be particularly intense and of longer duration, easily lasting three or four days and sometimes even longer. They are either present on awakening in the morning at severe intensity or wake the patient from sleep in the early morning hours, usually between four and six o'clock.

Both scenarios ask for powerful treatment, such as we can provide with the sumatriptan injection, ergotamine suppository, or dihydroergotamine injection. Due to sumatriptan's relatively short duration of action, the patient may need to repeat it for several consecutive days.

A good strategy is to decrease the intensity of the headache significantly with the sumatriptan injection, followed by the sumatriptan tablet to relieve it fully. Once fully alleviated, the headache generally remains controlled for approximately twenty-four hours, but it may be present again the next morning upon awakening. Then the patient should repeat the injection, tablet, or both depending on the intensity of the headache when they take the medication, always pursuing the treatment until the headache is fully relieved.

The advantage of using the ergotamine suppository or the dihydroergotamine injection is that as ergots, they have a long duration of action. Consequently, with a one- or two-day treatment, they may terminate a migraine headache in one or two days that would otherwise last three or four days.

When using an ergot, it is advisable to pretreat with an anti-nausea medication—for example, ten milligrams of metoclopramide or four milligrams of ondansetron by mouth fifteen minutes before—even if nausea is not present. If nausea is already present, we may have to administer the medications by intramuscular injection for good benefit.

The dose of dihydroergotamine is one milligram, and the ergotamine suppository generally contains two milligrams of the medication, along with one hundred milligrams of caffeine. The two-milligram dose in the suppository is often too much for migraineurs to tolerate because of nausea and vomiting. A suppository containing one milligram of the medication, along with one hundred milligrams of caffeine, is sometimes also available.

I always recommend that patients cut the two-milligram ergotamine suppository into thirds and take only a third at a time, if necessary, repeated every hour depending on the tolerability. They should repeat it until the headache is fully alleviated and may have to take additional medication the next morning if residual headache is present on awakening. It is prudent to cut the one-milligram ergotamine suppository into halves as well, take only a half at a time, and repeat it if necessary.

I have found migraine patients to be particularly sensitive to medications, and if side effects happen, it is difficult, if not impossible, to get them to use the medication again. Therefore, it is better to be on the safe side—start with as low a dose as is reasonable and repeat it with short enough intervals to obtain a cumulative benefit but at intervals that are long enough to prevent the occurrence of side effects.

While the menstrual cycle is by far the most potent trigger of headaches, including migraine headaches, affecting the majority of women with migraine, the most common headache triggers in general are stress, not eating on time, fatigue, and lack of sleep.

Of these four, not eating on time is undoubtedly the easiest to address by eating regularly during the day, preferably thrice, and not going without food too long, which includes fasting. In terms of preventing migraine headaches, it is probably more important that you eat regularly than what you eat. The latter means that I do not recommend dietary restrictions or migraine diets, because the benefit generally does not justify the effort or the expense often involved.

Insomnia

Regarding lack of sleep, it is important to realize that most people need eight or nine hours of uninterrupted sleep per night to feel well and function to their full capacity. If lack of sleep is due to lifestyle, it is crucial to change that by going to bed on time, because oversleeping in the morning can also trigger headache.

With eating and sleeping alike, regularity is key. Hence, eat at set times during the day, and do the same with sleeping; retire at night and arise in the morning at consistent times as well.

If lack of sleep is due to difficulties falling asleep, sleeping through the night, or waking up early, we need to address these issues. If all three are present, we call it primary insomnia, and the best treatment in my experience is with a medication called trazodone. This is a medication originally marketed for depression, but it is not very effective, to say the least, as an antidepressant.

Fluoxetine, the first selective serotonin reuptake inhibitor, or SSRI, is much more effective, but it can cause insomnia, for which we found the trazodone to be helpful. This led to its use for the treatment of primary insomnia in general, for which it is beneficial although it is not a sleeping medication.

Sleeping medications, also called hypnotics, have the disadvantage of potentially being addictive and making sleep dependent on them, which means that after some time, it becomes difficult to sleep without them. Trazodone does not have this downside, and in addition, patients generally tolerate it well without side effects.

If falling asleep is a problem, the patient should take the medication approximately two hours before bedtime, because it takes time for it to get absorbed into the body and cause drowsiness. If drowsiness is still present on awakening the next morning, the dose is too high, and finding the right one may take some time.

A good starting dose is 25 or 50 milligrams but even this may be too high, and we can certainly initiate treatment with one as low as 12.5 milligrams. We should slowly increase it, allowing enough time to assess efficacy and tolerability in terms of daytime drowsiness.

The ultimate goal is to secure eight or nine hours of uninterrupted sleep per night and feeling refreshed, not groggy, on awakening in the morning.

The usual dose to accomplish this lies somewhere between 50 and 150 milligrams, but it can be as low as 12.5 or 25 milligrams or as high as 300 or 400 milligrams. The absolute dose is not important, however; what is relevant is that we secure adequate, good sleep without causing daytime drowsiness. After all, the ultimate goal is to improve daytime fatigue, and lack of sleep is often the culprit.

Falling Asleep

If the sleeping difficulty is limited to falling asleep, the question we should ask is what prevents the person from falling asleep. Is it racing thoughts, an inability to get comfortable in bed, or restlessness of the legs with an irresistible urge to move them?

If the problem is an inability to get comfortable in bed, it may be due to something that we can address, like discomfort or pain. In case of racing thoughts, a relatively fast- and short-acting sedating medication, like gabapentin, may be helpful. Here, it may take some time as well to find the right dose, which can lie anywhere between one hundred and six hundred to nine hundred milligrams, taken at or shortly before bedtime.

If the issue is tightness or soreness of the neck, shoulder, and upper back muscles, a common problem especially in patients with chronic migraine, the use of a heating pad before bedtime may provide solace. In those patients, I recommend the daily use of heat anyway, preferably upon rising in the morning and retiring at night, each time for fifteen to twenty minutes. Using a heating pad on a daily basis will, in due time, reduce the tightness and soreness of the muscles, often with benefit on the headaches as well.

If the difficulty falling asleep is due to restlessness of the legs with an irresistible urge to move them, we are dealing with restless legs syndrome, or RLS. In my experience, the best treatment is with a small dose of a medication for Parkinson's disease called pramipexole taken at dinnertime and at bedtime. I usually prescribe

0.125 milligram for each intake but may increase the dose to 0.25 milligram. Patients generally tolerate these dosages of the medication well without side effects.

If the problem falling asleep is associated with an inability to get up in the morning, it is likely that the issue is a delayed sleep phase disorder, as we call it. This is a condition very similar to experiencing a jet lag traveling east; you cannot fall asleep until one or two o'clock or later and cannot get up in the morning unless with great effort. In addition, despite eight or more hours of sleep, you end up feeling tired all day or even exhausted.

Delayed sleep phase disorder is something that we especially encounter in teenagers and adolescents, in my experience more often in boys than in girls, and is to a certain extent normal for that age. When severe, however, it significantly interferes with school attendance and school performance alike due to an inability to attend early classes and the extreme tiredness associated with it. The fatigue, in turn, easily leads to headaches, and when migraine runs in the family, these headaches are likely to be intense, further disabling the person.

Treatment is difficult, and apart from moving west or, when working, signing up for the three-to-eleven-o'clock shift, melatonin is your best bet. It is a hormone that regulates the night-day or sleep-wake cycle, also referred to as circadian rhythm. For melatonin to be helpful, however, the patient needs to take it with great regularity and at the right time. This means not just daily but every day at approximately the same time two hours before desired bedtime or sleep time. The dose does not seem to matter as long as it is immediate release, but the regularity and timing of intake matter a great deal.

Fatigue

Whether lack of sleep is due to lifestyle, primary insomnia, restless legs syndrome, delayed sleep phase disorder, or anything else for that matter, it causes fatigue. Fatigue to the extent that it is associated with sleeping long hours at night with additional hours napping during the day, we call hypersomnolence and suggests a problem with energy metabolism.

Further exploring this kind of fatigue, maybe better referred to as exhaustion, requires blood testing for low hemoglobin, or anemia; low iron reserve; low thyroid function, or hypothyroidism; and low vitamin B levels, particularly vitamin B_9, also called folate or folic acid, and vitamin B_{12}, also called cobalamin.

It is important to consider the results of blood tests in terms of what their optimum levels should be rather than whether they are within the reference ranges, often erroneously called normal values. When it comes to blood test results in general, we do not know what normal is, because we are not born with a manual in our hands. The laboratory performing the tests determines the so-called reference ranges, which are specific to that laboratory.

An optimum hemoglobin level for women is approximately 13.5 grams per deciliter (8.4 millimoles per liter), for men it is approximately 15 grams per deciliter (9.3 millimoles per liter), and the optimum level of iron reserve, ferritin, is sixty to eighty nanograms per milliliter.

With regard to thyroid function, we should measure the level of the thyroid-stimulating hormone, or TSH, in addition to that of the thyroid hormone levothyroxine, or T4. These levels should be in an inverse relation to each other, preferably with the free levothyroxine level, or FT4, relatively high and the thyroid-stimulating hormone level relatively low—for example, approximately 0.5 micro-international units per milliliter.

The recommended vitamin B_9 level is twenty nanograms per milliliter or higher, and the level of vitamin B_{12} should be at least three hundred picograms per milliliter.

Stress

Stress is a very different story and is generally difficult to tackle. It is a normal part of life but can be a problem when it is more than the person can shoulder, and this, of course, differs between individuals.

Chronic stress undermines physical and mental health and is important to deal with, preferably by addressing its cause or causes, however difficult that may be. The assistance of a therapist may be required to help with the stress and mitigate, if possible, its effects on physical and mental health and well-being.

A variety of relaxation and stress-coping exercises is available, but when employed, the patient should apply them consistently and on a daily basis. The one relaxation exercise that I do not recommend is progressive muscular relaxation, which requires forceful tightening of muscles followed by relaxing them. I have seen this technique bring on severe headaches in migraineurs when pressing the back of the head against the floor, causing the muscles in the back of the neck to go into spasm. Especially in patients with chronic migraine, these muscles are tight due to an inability to relax, and causing them to go into spasm makes the headaches worse.

The same is true for aggressive physical therapy directed at those muscles, which can be equally detrimental. Instead, I prefer the daily use of a heating pad and, if necessary, very gentle stretching exercises performed along with it and in one direction at a time only. However, the daily use of heat may suffice, provided the patient applies it every day—if possible, twice per day—for fifteen to twenty minutes each time.

Relaxation approaches that I particularly like are those derived from hypnotherapy, such as self-hypnosis, for example, with arm levitation. I also like imagery, but even simple breathing exercises, such as focusing on abdominal breathing, can be beneficial. The simpler the exercises, the better they are; the cheaper, the better as well.

For those kinds of exercises to be effective, they do not have to be expensive. However, they need to be practiced regularly for best benefit, preferably daily; if time permits and they are short, several times per day.

Diet

The question of diet often emerges in relation to migraine, but whatever it is, I have never seen it work. In addition, it is difficult to maintain them over time, especially over a long time, as is evident from the debacle of weight loss diets.

My general dietary advice for migraineurs is not to drink more than one or two cups of coffee per day, and if possible, to drink decaffeinated coffee only. I do not have an issue with tea because of its lower caffeine content, and the fact that people generally do not drink as much of it as they do coffee. Of course, what goes for coffee also applies to caffeinated sodas.

I also recommend migraineurs to be careful with alcohol, particularly red wine, especially when other triggers are present as well. However, the most important and most effective dietary advice, in my opinion, is to eat regularly, three meals per day.

Probably the worst-case scenario for bringing on a migraine headache is to go out for a drink on a Friday evening after work. The week may have been busy and stressful, having a drink delays dinner, late dinner defers bedtime, and Saturday morning is the time to sleep in, missing the first cup of coffee of the day. Multiple triggers potentially compound here to make a weekend migraine more likely than not to develop.

A migraine headache, when triggered by stress, typically occurs afterward, during the relaxation that follows; in this regard, it is more a relaxation headache than a stress headache. The greater the stress, the steeper the change in body physiology when relaxation finally happens and the more likely for a migraine headache to occur.

Add to that the fatigue from a busy week at work, going without food too long, alcohol, oversleeping, and caffeine withdrawal, that combined create the perfect scenario for the development of a migraine headache.

Compounding

What brings on a headache, migraine or otherwise, is often not a single trigger acting in solitude but, as in the example above, a compounding of triggers. Consequently, it is usually more effective and requires less of an effort to keep triggers from compounding rather than avoiding them.

However, we first need to identify them from the very long list of potential triggers, and a good way of doing so is for the patient to write down possible triggers each time a headache happens. It is best to do this after the headache, when the mind is clear again, asking oneself the question as to what, if anything, brought it on.

It is important to write down any thoughts that surface and not to rely on your memory, because it will fail you. Proceeding this way over time will generate a list of potential triggers, which will be long for most migraineurs.

The next step is to look at all of them and pick out half a dozen or so that are easiest to avoid without disrupting your lifestyle. You should try to eliminate those from your life, and with a little bit of luck, you will reduce the compounding of triggers to the extent that the frequency of your migraine headaches will go down.

Nose-Sinus System

In my experience, migraineurs are particularly sensitive to smells, pleasant or unpleasant, as triggers of their headaches and to weather changes, especially the decrease in barometric pressure with impending rain or snow. I mention them together because I think that both involve the nose-sinus system, which may be more important in migraine than generally assumed.

The underlying issue may be chronic, low-grade inflammation of the lining of the nose and sinuses. This, on the one hand, sensitizes the nerve fibers in the nose serving smell, which are the olfactory nerve fibers, causing smell sensitivity or osmophobia, also called odorphobia. On the other hand, it narrows the openings from the nose to the sinuses, which in some people are already narrow from birth—that is, congenitally.

If the latter is indeed the case, the additional narrowing may well be enough to close off the sinuses from the nose, making it difficult for them to adjust to changes in barometric pressure. Consequently, a pressure gradient develops over the sinuses when barometric pressure drops, causing the drawing midface pain typical of sinus headache. In migraineurs, such a pressure gradient puts stress, or strain, on the system, bringing about a migraine headache, with or without a sinus headache bridging the gap.

Nonseasonal allergies, such as to dust mites or animals, if around, most likely cause the aforementioned chronic, low-grade inflammation. Under such circumstances, we can do formal allergy testing, but I have never really found that helpful, possibly because negative findings do not mean anything, and positive findings may not be relevant.

If there is suspicion of allergic rhinitis—or allergic rhinosinusitis, to be more precise—initiating treatment makes more sense to see whether it renders a difference in headache occurrence. The allergy treatment that I prefer is with an intranasal antihistamine, such as azelastine, dosed one spray four times per day. An alternative is a medication called cromolyn, which is a so-called mast cell stabilizer, also in a dose of one spray four times per day. Mast cells are the source of the histamine in the lining of the nose and sinuses released with allergies, causing the inflammation.

Prodromes

Discussing headache triggers brings us to the confusing area of migraine prodromes, which are the generally vague complaints that may precede migraine headaches by hours or days. They are different from migraine aura, which presents with well-defined neurological symptoms, mostly visual in nature, occurring over well-defined times, usually lasting fifteen to thirty minutes.

Prodromal complaints, among others, include yawning, fatigue, irritability, anxiety, difficulty concentrating, feeling cold, being down in the dumps, sweet craving, light sensitivity, blurred vision, muscle tightness, and nausea. Many of them can also accompany migraine headaches as associated symptoms or even follow them, when we call them postdromes.

Does it make sense to look at prodromal and postdromal complaints when it comes to migraine? As far as I am concerned, not to a great extent and certainly not when it relates to postdromes, which likely result from inadequate treatment of the headache, from not addressing whatever brought it on, or from something else going on medically.

On the other hand, examining prodromal symptoms may provide at least some insight into what brings on the headaches. However, when analyzing them in terms of triggers, it is important to realize that some of them belong together and have a common origin.

Fatigue, a very important one and, as far as I am concerned, the biological trigger of headache, comes along with yawning, irritability, difficulty concentrating, feeling cold, sweet craving, and muscle tightness. The reason it occurs with sweet craving is because carbohydrates constitute the quickest and energetically cheapest way of making metabolic energy. Muscles need energy to relax and with fatigue, when metabolic energy is in short supply, relaxation is inadequate, and muscles remain tight.

Feeling cold with fatigue is the body's effort to preserve heat by narrowing, or constricting, the blood vessels in the distal parts, particularly in the hands and feet, referred to as acra. It is very much like what we do at home in the winter: during the day, we turn off the heaters in the bedrooms to preserve heat and keep the living area nice and warm.

Other complaints that go together are sensitivity to light, or photophobia, and blurred vision, the latter particularly of near vision. When those symptoms happen before the onset of the headache, they suggest eyestrain as a potential trigger.

Eyestrain occurs when the muscles of accommodation, which are the little muscles in the eyes that surround the lenses, are relatively weak. When these muscles, which are also called ciliary muscles, contract, the lenses become rounder and bring anything up close into focus. The opposite happens when they relax and the lenses become flatter, allowing for in-focus distant vision.

When the muscles of accommodation are relatively weak and used intensely—for example, with prolonged reading or working at a computer monitor—they tire and give way. When this occurs, it makes vision blurred, especially near vision, and the eyes become sensitive to light, or photophobic. The latter happens because the eyes cope with light in the same way they allow for near vision, namely by contracting the muscles of accommodation.

The remedy is to interrupt the reading or working at a computer monitor regularly and relax the muscles of accommodation by staring into the distance, preferably out of a window. It is equally important to perform those activities in a well-lighted environment, preferably lit by incandescent light. Making the font bigger and the contrast lower are also ways of addressing eyestrain, as well as employing low-strength magnifiers—for example, 0.5 or 1 diopter reading glasses.

For coping with bright light, sunglasses with green-glass lenses are ideal. Green impacts visual acuity less than brown while being equally effective in protecting the eyes against bright light. Plastic, as opposed to glass, distorts vision, which is an additional strain to the eyes. This is especially important if the sunglasses are worn often, which a person who is generally sensitive to light should certainly do.

Gastritis

Nausea preceding or following migraine headaches—that is, occurring as a prodrome or postdrome—or happening with relatively mild headaches suggests the presence of a stomach problem, particularly gastritis. This is a chronic, low-grade inflammation of the lining of the stomach, which apart from nausea can cause pain in the stomach area, heartburn, or reflux. The stomach area is the part of the abdomen immediately below the breastbone, which we also refer to as epigastric area.

It is a condition caused by the retention of acid due to slow stomach emptying, allowing the acid to irritate the lining of the stomach and render it inflamed. The inflammation, in turn, leads to tiny ulcerations that cause chronic blood loss in the stool, ultimately giving rise to low hemoglobin, or anemia, and iron deficiency.

In and of itself, nausea is probably not a headache trigger; in publications, however, I have described reflux as a trigger of migraine headaches. Many, if not most, processes in biology and medicine are circular rather than linear, and this is the case with headaches as well, especially with intense headaches like migraine.

Intense headaches make the neck, shoulder, and upper back muscles tight; the tightness, in turn, increases the frequency and intensity of the headaches. The same is true with the stomach, because intense headaches retard its emptying, causing retention of acid, which in turn brings on headaches.

There are many other examples of circular relations in biology and medicine, even just related to migraine, with the advantage that circles offer many options for intervention or treatment.

Mentor

Related to headache triggers, my mentor, John R. Graham, in a book titled *Treatment of Migraine*, published in 1955 by Little, Brown, & Company, wrote the following about errors in living:

> Presented below is a list of common deviations from hygienic living in which many persons may well indulge with impunity but that are frequently a source of headache to the sufferer from migraine. Behind these errors in living, lie attitudes in the patient that serve both to bring them about and to intensify the damage they create. Such errors may have to be arbitrarily eliminated at first, but as treatment progresses it is fundamental to ultimate success for the patient to gain insight into his attitudes and personality

traits that brought them about and to attempt suitable alteration. The errors are as follows:

- Poor meals—skimpy breakfasts and lunches and large dinners eaten in a state of fatigue.
- Irregular hours for meals. Postponing lunch for an hour may give anyone a mild headache, but may produce a bad sick headache for the migraine patient.
- Morning deadlines. Too little time is allowed between the rising hour and the scramble for school and office.
- Sleeping late on Saturdays, Sundays and holidays. The patient with migraine needs a good deal of sleep—but not in the morning. Conversely, getting to bed early is important, since, to date, the only real cure for fatigue is rest.
- Lack of breaks in the day. A short rest in the morning and afternoon, regularly obtained, is helpful.
- Overcrowded schedules. Patients usually try to work in too many events in a day. They need to spread their activities more evenly over several days.
- Failure to take proper vacations.
- Failure to get away from their children periodically.
- Excessive participation in community and church activities.
- Overanxiety regarding preparations for guests, shopping trips and vacations.
- Long automobile trips. The migraine patient usually wishes to go the five

hundred miles in one day and ends up with a headache.

- Acting as chair (because nobody else will accept). Migraine patients do not delegate work to others. They do it all themselves.
- Making up for lost time. As soon as the patients are over one attack, they usually rush to repair the losses. Consequently, the next attack comes sooner.
- Suffering petty wrongs in silence until they mount to unbearable heights. It would be better to settle differences while they are small.
- Aiming for impossible goals and worrying when they cannot be attained.
- Lack of exercise.
- Lack of recreation.

Chapter 10

What about My General Health?

Chronic Migraine

General health, mental and physical, is usually not a problem in migraineurs with relatively infrequent headaches, a presentation that we have come to refer to as episodic migraine. This is almost always different in those with frequent headaches, whom we now consider to suffer from chronic migraine. We look at the difference between the two in terms of the overall headache frequency, which I like to refer to as the total headache burden.

With episodic migraine, officially, the total headache burden is less than half a month; with chronic migraine, it is half a month or more. Of course, there is nothing magical about half a month, making the distinction between the two based on overall headache frequency arbitrary and, hence, devoid of biological or medical significance. The picture becomes different, however, when we consider the presentations in light of the general health of those afflicted; their health tends to be good in episodic migraineurs and relatively poor in chronic migraineurs.

People often develop chronic migraine over time, and although this is by far not always the case, I used to believe that those with chronic migraine come down with their relatively poor general health over time as well, maybe even because of the headaches. Mainly due to seeing younger patients with chronic migraine, especially teenagers and adolescents, I arrived at a different view on this vexing problem.

Before I delve into this any further, however, let me present some examples of the presentation of chronic migraine as I have seen it in practice. I have selected patients of an age range to demonstrate that there is no age-dependent difference, which translates into a difference due to length of migraine suffering.

An eighteen-year-old woman has been experiencing migraine since the age of eleven; she started menstruating at age twelve. The headaches occur daily and usually come on during the day, but not at any particular time. They are moderately severe in intensity (7–8/10) and severe (9–10/10), once or twice per week for one or two days.

The headaches are located in the forehead, eyes, temples, and back of the head. They are throbbing in nature, and physical activity makes them worse. The headaches are associated with light and noise sensitivity and, when severe, with nausea as well.

Apart from the headaches, she has insomnia and gets, on average, five hours of sleep per night. As a result, she feels tired during the day and rates her energy level as a two on a ten-point scale. She also has anxiety, depression, and attention deficit disorder. She has reflux and diarrhea-predominant irritable bowel syndrome; she used to be constipated. Her neck and shoulder muscles are tight and sore.

A twenty-eight-year-old woman has been experiencing migraine since the age of thirteen; she started menstruating at age twelve. The headaches happen almost daily and are often present on awakening in the morning at moderate intensity (5/10). In approximately half, they worsen as the day progresses to become severe (8/10) by early afternoon; otherwise, they remain moderate.

The headaches involve the entire head but, when severe, concentrate in the left forehead and behind the left eye. They are throbbing in nature, and physical activity makes them worse. The headaches are associated with light and noise sensitivity and, when severe, also with nausea and, twice per month on average, with vomiting as well.

Apart from the headaches, she has insomnia and gets, on average, six or seven hours of interrupted sleep per night. As a result, she feels tired during the day and rates her energy level as a six on a ten-point scale.

She has depression and irritable bowel syndrome, alternating between diarrhea and constipation. Her periods occur twice per month, last seven days, and are heavy and very painful. Her neck and shoulder muscles are tight and sore, and she has had low back pain since childhood.

A forty-three-year-old woman has been experiencing migraine since the age of sixteen; she started menstruating at age fifteen. The headaches have been severe (8–9/10) since their onset, associated with nausea and blurred vision. Initially, they happened once per week but, due to a gradual increase in frequency, they have been daily since the age of thirty-seven.

The daily headaches come on late morning and increase in intensity as the day progresses. They are moderately severe in intensity (7/10) and severe (8–9/10) twice per week for one or two days. The severe headaches develop during the day and reach their maximum intensity in half an hour.

The headaches are located across the forehead and in the back of the head. They are throbbing in nature, and physical activity makes them worse. The headaches never occur or worsen in relation to the menstrual cycle. Her periods have always been infrequent, short, and light but very painful. She had a hysterectomy at the age of thirty-six because of painful intercourse and has had night sweats since.

At the age of thirty, she began experiencing pain in her neck, shoulders, upper back, and lower back, which worsened over time. Subsequently, it extended into her extremities, leading to the diagnosis of fibromyalgia. At the same time, she started having problems falling asleep and sleeping through the night, resulting in fatigue.

At the age of thirty-three, she developed irritable bowel syndrome with constipation and diarrhea. Two or three times per week, she does not have a bowel movement for one or two days and then develops a cramping pain in her lower abdomen. Invariably within ten minutes of eating, she has two or three bowel movements with improvement of the pain. The movements start with hard stool, followed by diarrhea or watery stool.

At the age of thirty-seven, she was found to have high blood pressure, resulting in the diagnosis of hypertension. At the age of thirty-

eight, she developed pain in her jaws, worse on the right than on the left, progressive over time. At the same age, her nose became chronically congested, supposedly from allergies.

At the age of thirty-nine, she developed daily nausea while previously she had only experienced it with the severe headaches. The daily nausea is associated with heartburn, but not with stomach pain or reflux.

The following is a listing of potential conditions seen in association with chronic migraine—in this context, disorders that we refer to as comorbidities of chronic migraine:

- Anxiety
- Chronic nausea
- Reflux, or GERD
- Constipation
- Depression
- Chronic fatigue
- Widespread body pain, or fibromyalgia
- Difficulty sleeping, or insomnia
- Irritable bowel syndrome, or IBS
- Low back pain, or lumbago
- Menstrual cycle disorders, such as infrequent menstruation, or oligomenorrhea; frequent menstruation, or polymenorrhea; and irregular menstrual cycle
- Menstruation disorders, such as heavy menstruation, called hypermenorrhea or menorrhagia; and painful menstruation, or dysmenorrhea
- Neck pain, or cervicalgia
- Temporomandibular disorder, or TMD

Comorbidities

I am sure that the above list is not complete, but it certainly covers most of the medical and psychiatric conditions regularly encountered in patients with chronic migraine. We generally refer to them as comorbid disorders, or comorbidities, meaning additional conditions occurring with a primary one—in this case, chronic migraine.

Comorbidities may be a chance occurrence, may have developed due to a shared cause, may be the result of another comorbid condition, or may be caused by a third and unknown ailment. We often assume that they are independent of the primary disorder and without impact on it. However, particularly when it comes to chronic migraine, this may not be the case, as I will come back to later.

In the past, we considered the comorbidities merely in choosing preventive migraine treatment, hoping that the preventive medication treats the particular comorbid condition as well. Examples of this are the use of propranolol for migraine prevention when high blood pressure, or hypertension, is an issue as well, the prescribing of amitriptyline when insomnia is present, or the use of topiramate when we aim at mood stabilization for the patient.

I consider this approach old-fashioned, because we can now expect more benefit on the primary disorder as well as on the comorbid conditions from specific medications. The employment of specific medications is key, whether it is for the abortive or preventive treatment of migraine or for the treatment of any other disorder, comorbid with migraine or not. When a physician or other health care practitioner prescribes a nonspecific medication for any condition, migraine or otherwise, it is important to inquire as to the rationale.

The specific medications for abortive migraine treatment are the ergots, triptans, and gepants. We should not use the ergots for migraine abortion unless there is a particular reason. For preventive migraine treatment, the specific medications are beta-blockers, gepants, and CGRP antibodies. When prescribing a medication out of the class of beta-blockers, we should avoid propranolol because of its generally poor tolerability.

Anxiety and Depression

Anxiety and depression are common comorbidities of migraine, but we see them much more often with chronic migraine than with episodic migraine. We usually assume that the unpredictability of occurrence of migraine headaches and their disabling nature cause anxiety, which in turn leads to depression. This is certainly true, but it may not be the whole story.

In fact, studies suggest that anxiety precedes the onset of migraine, and depression follows it. At the same time, anxiety may further increase the frequency of migraine headaches, and depression may make it more difficult to cope with them. This is just one example of how complicated it gets and how entangled patients can become in a web of diagnoses and treatments, from which it is difficult to escape.

There are numerous treatments available for anxiety and depression, ranging from counseling and psychotherapy to medications. A first and relatively simple step in the right direction is to consider relaxation exercises, of which there is a large number available and of various kinds. It is important to find the one that you really like, because they only work if practiced regularly, preferably daily.

In addition, the exercise needs to be simple and easy to learn without requiring a gadget—or anything else, for that matter. Probably the simplest relaxation exercise is to take a moment and focus on abdominal breathing, which you can do not just daily but many times during the day. It is simple, physical, does not require a lot of concentration, and is easy to do when feeling particularly anxious.

Controlling anxiety improves depression, if mild, because the two walk hand in hand like brother and sister. If either one is more than mild, we should seek additional measures, such as counseling, medication treatment, or both. We have a plethora of medications for the treatment of anxiety and depression, and we should use them when indicated.

I have observed that migraineurs generally do not tolerate medications well that have a stimulatory effect on the body. I came to realize this in the late eighties when the antidepressant fluoxetine was in development, and I consulted patients with headaches as a side effect of it.

These patients found the medication very helpful and, consequently, did not want to discontinue it. Given the nature of their headaches, I treated them successfully with one of the beta-blockers known to be effective for migraine prevention. A low dose generally sufficed, and I avoided propranolol because of its relatively high likelihood of making depression worse.

I found the next antidepressant that came around, sertraline, much better tolerated, and it has remained my treatment of choice for anxiety and depression, especially in migraineurs. Of course, when either one is severe, more advanced treatments are required; as far as I am concerned, it is still better to avoid stimulating medications, however. This also applies to the treatment of attention deficit disorder, or ADD, and we should never prescribe them for the treatment of fatigue per se.

In medicine, we often consider fatigue a depression-related symptom, and it certainly can be. However, before labeling it as such, we should always first investigate it for common medical causes, like low hemoglobin, or anemia, iron deficiency, and low thyroid function, or hypothyroidism.

Insomnia

Along with anxiety and depression, fatigue is almost invariably present in patients with chronic migraine, and it is generally of a chronic nature. Although often comorbid with depression, it should only be ascribed to it after thorough evaluation, medical and otherwise. Probably the most common reason for fatigue in the chronic migraineur is comorbid insomnia.

The insomnia is generally of the primary type with problems falling asleep, sleeping through the night, and waking up early. It is important to treat it, also in the context of treating anxiety and depression, which are unlikely to improve if we allow the insomnia to persist. In general, however, we should not treat it with sleeping medications, called hypnotics, because they will render the sleep dependent on them and, over time, make matters worse.

A good medication for the treatment of primary insomnia is trazodone, itself an antidepressant but not a very effective one and, consequently, rarely prescribed anymore for this indication. It gained popularity for the treatment of insomnia when fluoxetine became available, and we realized that the latter commonly causes insomnia.

Patients generally tolerate the trazodone well, without side effects, and they can use it long-term for insomnia without any problems. A good alternative is gabapentin, especially when falling asleep is an issue, because it is short-acting.

If falling asleep is the only problem and the patient sleeps well through the night, we should consider the possibilities of restless legs syndrome, or RLS, and delayed sleep phase disorder. With the latter, it is difficult rising in the morning as well, similar to when we are jet-lagged traveling east. It is not easy to treat, but we can try immediate-release melatonin, taken daily in a very consistent manner, approximately two hours before retiring.

An irresistible urge to move the legs characterizes restless legs syndrome, usually upon lying down in bed to sleep. However, it may already start in the evening upon sitting down to relax or watch television. The restlessness can be so intense that it forces the patient to get up from sitting or lying down and pace the floor, generally without much relief. The best treatment, in my experience, is with a medication marketed for Parkinson's disease called pramipexole. Generally, a small dose will do, and I like to start it already at dinnertime, giving 0.125 or 0.25 milligram then and the same dose at bedtime.

Fatigue

The medical evaluation of fatigue requires blood tests to determine the levels of hemoglobin, ferritin, vitamin B_9 (folate or folic acid), vitamin B_{12} (cobalamin), thyroid-stimulating hormone (TSH), and free levothyroxine (FT4).

The hemoglobin serves to diagnose anemia, and the level should be approximately 13.5 grams per deciliter in women (8.4 millimoles per liter) and approximately 15 grams per deciliter in men (9.3 millimoles per liter).

The ferritin level determines the iron reserve and should be at least sixty to eighty nanograms per milliliter in women of childbearing potential. However, I like to see it at that approximate level for all women and consider it a good value for men as well.

Energy metabolism needs B vitamins, particularly vitamin B_9, folate or folic acid, and vitamin B_{12}, cobalamin, and their levels should be at least twenty nanograms per milliliter and three hundred picograms per milliliter respectively.

Regarding thyroid function, we should not only determine the level of the thyroid-stimulating hormone, or TSH, as is often done, but also that of free levothyroxine, or FT4. Ideally, the results of these two hormones should be such that they are in an inverse relation to each other, with the levothyroxine level relatively high in relation to the reference range and the thyroid-stimulating hormone level relatively low.

I do not remember ever having seen both levels high in relation to the reference ranges, but I have certainly observed both on the low side. As far as I am concerned, this is abnormal, and I will further evaluate it by prescribing a small dose of levothyroxine, usually fifty micrograms per day, and retest after six to eight weeks. This should increase the levothyroxine level and bring the thyroid-stimulating hormone level further down.

However, I have also seen a small amount of levothyroxine increase the thyroid-stimulating hormone level, which is an abnormal response. In such cases, I will gradually further increase the dose until the levothyroxine level in the blood is relatively high and the thyroid-stimulating hormone level has gone down again, creating an inverse relation between the two as I like it to be.

Of course, in the meantime, I monitor the level of fatigue and make sure that my efforts result in a decrease in fatigue and an improvement in energy level, the ultimate goal of the treatment.

Muscle Tightness

Along with fatigue, which is due to a lack of metabolic energy and probably because of it, the muscles of a chronic migraineur, the postural ones in particular, are tight. The latter are the muscles that keep us upright, and as we are erect beings, they require more energy than our movement muscles.

Contrary to what people generally think, muscles do not need energy to contract but to relax. Without the necessary energy, they cannot relax and, hence, remain tight; in case of the postural muscles, tightness of the neck, shoulders, upper back, lower back, and calves develops.

Continuous, or persistent, tightness or soreness of neck, shoulder, and upper back muscles is invariably present in chronic migraine patients. It drives headache frequency and, to a certain extent, also headache intensity, which I base on my extensive experience treating those patients with botulinum toxin.

The chronic muscle tightness, which exists in the head as well but is less perceptible there because of a lack of joints, is the treatment target of botulinum toxin. It is often also present in the jaw muscles, which are not postural muscles but align with them so that our mouth does not drop open whenever we stand up.

The condition that results from the chronic tightness of the jaw muscles is known as temporomandibular disorder, or TMD. People often erroneously refer to it as TMJ, but that acronym stands for *temporomandibular joint*, which is the joint that you can feel in front of the ear when you open and close your mouth.

Treatment with botulinum toxin is very effective for temporomandibular disorder and, in my experience, more so for this condition than it is for chronic migraine. We administer it quarterly, and while the benefit lasts shorter in chronic migraine, it may persist for three to six months or even longer in temporomandibular disorder. In this condition, we can use it by itself or in combination with an oral appliance, which is the standard treatment to prevent clenching and grinding, called bruxism, and very importantly, to protect the structure of the teeth as well.

For the tightness of the neck, shoulder, and upper back muscles, I recommend the daily use of a heating pad for fifteen to twenty minutes each time. With its consistent application, we will see a gradual reduction in muscle tightness over weeks or months. For this purpose, I like the microwavable heating pad better than the electric one, because it provides moist heat, which penetrates better.

Heat does not penetrate well in general, which is why taking a hot shower or a hot bath does not suffice. It also means that it requires good contact—for example, by lying on the heating pad or by sitting in a high-back chair with the heating pad between the body and the back of the chair.

Gentle massage is an option as well, but added to the daily use of the heating pad and not instead of it. It needs to be gentle, however, not to make the headaches worse, which can easily happen when applied too forcefully. If you add stretching, you should do this very carefully as well and only in one direction at a time, as opposed to rolling the head around.

While stretching to the side, you should take care not to overstretch, and I prefer any treatment not to include this kind of exercise. Stretching the back of the neck you can easily accomplish by bending the neck forward or by tucking the chin back. You can do this during the daily application of the heating pad, which you can also combine with a general relaxation exercise.

The relaxation exercise that I do not recommend is progressive muscular relaxation. It requires vigorously contracting muscles before relaxing them, and contracting the muscles in the back of the neck, especially against a hard surface like the floor, can make them go into spasm and cause severe headache.

If the muscle tightness affects the calf muscles, it can cause cramps, especially at night, for which I have found vitamin B_1, or thiamine, to be beneficial in a dose of one hundred milligrams per day.

Gut Muscles

It is my impression that the problem with muscle relaxation as it impacts the postural muscles can also affect the smooth muscles in the gut. When these muscles do not relax as well as they should, it renders the forward movement of the gut, its propulsive activity, slow. This forward moving activity, also called peristalsis, empties the stomach, moves the stool through the small bowel, and empties the large bowel.

With slow peristalsis, the stomach does not empty out well and retains acid that generates complaints of nausea, heartburn, reflux, or stomach pain. When the large bowel, or colon, does not empty out well, constipation ensues with infrequent bowel movements and hard stool that requires straining to evacuate.

When the stomach irritation caused by the acid, known as gastritis, is particularly severe, it excessively stimulates the so-called gastrocolic reflex. This reflex, as the name implies, connects the stomach (*gaster* in Greek) with the large bowel (*colon* in Latin); its excessive stimulation leads to a disorder known as restaurant syndrome or to straightforward diarrhea. Restaurant syndrome is an urge to have a bowel movement and, consequently, the need to use the restroom immediately after consuming a meal, especially when heavy.

The constipation resulting from the slow emptying of the large bowel can lead to diarrhea, which indicates a worsening of the condition. This diarrhea is different from the one aforementioned, which I referred to as straightforward diarrhea, because it alternates with constipation, or with not having a bowel movement at all.

A pattern may subsequently develop in which a bowel movement does not occur for two or three days or longer, followed by bloating and lower abdominal pain. The pain often consists of wrenching cramps, and the diarrhea that follows can be explosive. When the bowel movement eases the bloating and abdominal pain, we refer to the disorder as irritable bowel syndrome, in this case of the mixed type, or IBS-M.

The diarrhea that happens with mixed irritable bowel syndrome we call paradoxical, because the underlying condition is constipation. It is the body's attempt to mitigate the problem by building up diarrhea behind the constipation with the ultimate goal of moving the hard stool to the point of evacuation.

Under those circumstances, it is important to ascertain that, along with the diarrhea, you do indeed evacuate hard stool. Otherwise, a vicious cycle develops in which the diarrhea passes by the constipation, and there is no progress, just suffering. The treatment is paradoxical as well, which means with a stool softener, laxative, or both, because it is, after all, constipation based.

If the diarrhea is due to excessive stimulation of the gastrocolic reflex because of gastritis, we should treat that instead. We have several classes of medications to do so, of which the proton-pump inhibitors, or PPIs, are by far the most effective.

However, we also have so-called H_2 blockers that we can employ, in which the *H* stands for *histamine*, such as cimetidine and famotidine, as well as medications to coat the stomach, like sucralfate. Patients generally tolerate them well without side effects, but I prefer the proton-pump inhibitors because of their potency.

Despite their strength, however, it is important that the patient takes them in a high enough dose and for a sufficiently long period. Dosing should be twice per day, preferably before breakfast and dinner, but if skipped at any of those times, it can be taken anytime.

If the dose is high enough, relief of symptoms ensues in one to two weeks or sooner, but that does not mean that we have solved the problem. It may take six to twelve months or longer for gastritis to heal, requiring the intake of the medication for that long.

What I encounter all the time with the use of a proton-pump inhibitor for the treatment of gastritis is that the dose is too low and, therefore, does not provide benefit or does not fully alleviate the complaints. Also, patients often discontinue it as soon as symptom relief occurs, not realizing that while they are feeling better, the underlying disorder is still present. They wonder why their complaints recur after stopping the medication and do not realize that symptom relief does not equate recovery from a condition.

If the proton-pump inhibitor in a relatively high dose is not fully effective, I add sucralfate, one gram taken before lunch and at bedtime. This is not really a medication, because it does not go anywhere but the stomach and does not get absorbed into the body. It coats the stomach and helps the healing of the irritation and, hence, the inflammation of its lining by binding the acid.

However, sucralfate binds not only the acid but anything consumed with it. Therefore, we should not take it together with other medications. If prescribed by itself to treat gastritis, the dose is one gram four times per day taken before meals and at bedtime.

In the context of migraine management, it is paramount to treat gastritis and constipation, if present, and this is as important as treating comorbid insomnia, for example. Treating those disorders may, like treating insomnia, improve the frequency and intensity of the migraine headaches.

If it does not improve the headaches, it will definitely contribute to the patient's overall well-being and, therefore, to their ability to cope with the headaches, mentally and physically. It may also ameliorate the impact of the migraine headaches, for example, on the stomach, which may not get upset as much, if not affected by gastritis. Treating gastritis invariably decreases the association of headaches with nausea and vomiting, even if it does not affect the headaches per se.

Below are examples of migraine patients who had reflux from gastritis and constipation respectively as comorbid disorders, treatment of which improved their overall migraine condition. I added a third example of a migraineur in whom indigestion was a major headache trigger.

Indigestion is also known as upset stomach or dyspepsia, and consists of an uncomfortable feeling of fullness shortly into the meal, called early satiety, with or without discomfort or pain in the stomach area. It is another example of how gastritis can present itself and relates directly to what causes it, which is the slow emptying of the stomach with the retention of acid.

With indigestion, however, the problem is not the acid but the food that is retained; in the patient vignette below, it is probably what was ingested during the day that made the stomach unable to tolerate even a small amount of additional food at night. A medication called metoclopramide, taken before dinner, effectively treated the indigestion and prevented the headaches from occurring.

Metoclopramide is an effective anti-nausea medication that, in addition to treating nausea, has the unique ability to stimulate the emptying of the stomach. The only other anti-nausea medication that does the same is domperidone. Anti-nausea medications in general retard stomach emptying and, therefore, are not great in the context of abortive migraine treatment when the emptying of the stomach is already slow due to the headache.

Patient Vignettes

The following are examples of migraine headaches associated with reflux, constipation, and indigestion respectively as comorbid disorders that negatively affected the frequency of headache occurrence:

A forty-three-year-old man has been experiencing migraine since the age of nineteen. The headaches happen four to eight times per month, usually lasting a day but sometimes two or three. Approximately half of them are present on awakening in the morning, especially with lack of sleep.

The headaches are generally located on the right, in the temple and in the eye, but sometimes on the left. They are moderate in intensity on awakening and become severe if not treated effectively. The headaches are always associated with nausea. When severe, they are also associated with vomiting and with congestion of the nostril on the side of the pain. Sumatriptan, fifty milligrams taken by mouth, generally provides full relief of the headaches within an hour.

When coming on during the day, the headaches tend to be on the left, extending from the cheek to the eye. His throat is often sore on the left, worse in the evening. He has had reflux for years with severe pain behind the breastbone but controlled with omeprazole, twenty milligrams once daily. Increasing the dose to twenty milligrams twice daily relieved the left throat soreness and abolished the left-sided headaches.

A forty-seven-year-old woman has been experiencing migraine since the age of twelve, when she started menstruating. Initially, the headaches occurred once every two months. Over time, they gradually increased in frequency and currently happen four to six times per month. The headaches occur consistently perimenstrually and then last two or three days; otherwise, they mostly last a day.

The headaches are usually present on awakening in the morning. They are located across the forehead and are dull, steady in nature. Sometimes, the headaches are located on the left only, in the forehead and behind the eye. They are associated with mild nausea, but not with light or noise sensitivity.

When mild or moderate in intensity, five milligrams of zolmitriptan with five hundred milligrams of naproxen consistently relieve the headaches fully. Sumatriptan, six milligrams administered by injection, fully abolishes them when severe.

She attributes approximately half of the headaches to constipation, which she has had for years with hard stool that is difficult to evacuate. She can count on waking up with headache when she has not had a bowel movement for three days. Treatment with magnesium citrate, four hundred milligrams per day, softened the stool and allowed almost daily movements, resolving the constipation-related headaches.

A fifty-year-old man has been experiencing migraine since early adulthood. The headaches happen at the night and wake him from sleep around three o'clock in the morning. They are severe and generally last until late afternoon. The headaches are located across the forehead and on top of the head, where they are throbbing in nature. They are associated with nausea and, when severe, also with vomiting.

Initially, only eating excessively late at night brought on the headaches. This was especially the case when he ate spicy food or black olives. However, the situation has been worse for the last two years. He now develops headaches during the night whenever he eats anything, even a snack, after nine o'clock in the evening. The later he eats, the more he eats, and the spicier the food, the more likely a headache will awake him.

He can sometimes prevent their occurrence after eating at night by taking a walk. Drinking carbonated soda to make him belch or taking an antacid with acetaminophen at bedtime is also helpful. He has had heartburn with a tendency to belch for many years, worse over time. Treatment with metoclopramide, ten milligrams taken before dinner, almost completely resolved the nocturnal headaches.

Metabolic Energy

With regard to the comorbidities of chronic migraine, the question arises as to whether they comprise a random collection of disorders. I do not believe that this is the case, but then how do they relate to each other, and how do they connect to chronic migraine? As I will explain later, I do think that they tie to chronic migraine but they are not part of it, as others have suggested.

Migraine is a genetically determined and inherited vulnerability to intense headaches, and it does not matter whether the condition is episodic or chronic. As far as I am concerned, it does not extend beyond that; in my opinion, migraine is not a disease, neurological or otherwise. However, many different factors influence its presentation, and when it comes to chronic migraine, this is where the comorbidities enter the picture.

The comorbidities do not constitute a random collection of disorders that chronic migraineurs accumulate over time. Their unifying factor, I think, is a lack of metabolic energy, which manifests itself in fatigue and is the biological reason we get headaches, although numerous other causes bring them on as well.

The biological reason refers to why we experience headaches to begin with and why they even exist—why there is such a thing as headache. However, the fatigue that directly relates to headache in this way is intermittent, or episodic, and leads to headache when ignored. The fatigue that is part of the comorbidities of chronic migraine is persistent, or chronic, accounting for the invariably chronic nature of the comorbid disorders associated with it.

Fatigue means a lack of metabolic energy, which is the energy that every one of the trillions of cells in our body requires for proper functioning. The energy is in the food that we eat, but for our cells to use it, the body needs to convert it into what we refer to as metabolic energy. It turns nutrients like carbohydrates and fats into metabolic energy in little energy factories inside the cells called mitochondria.

These little energy factories, or mitochondria, used to be independently living bacteria. They made their way into cells some 1.5 billion years ago in order to provide the cells with the energy required to function. They have their own genetic material which, like that of bacteria, is circular in nature, and we inherit it solely from the mother.

The mitochondria reside in the cell plasma which, during conception, comes from the mother, along with half of the cell nucleus; the other half comes from the father. Their genetic material, however, change or mutates easily, making it always slightly different from that of the mother.

When there is a shortage of metabolic energy, the focus of energy supply turns to the so-called vital organs, such as the brain, heart, lungs, kidneys, and liver. This leaves out some very large organs, such as the skin, the largest organ of our body; the skeletal muscles, which maintain our erect posture, allow us to move around, and physically protect our vital organs; and also the gut.

It is probably the regulation of thyroid function at the organ level that accomplishes this redistribution of metabolic energy. The impact of it is especially noticeable when it comes to the muscles, particularly the skeletal muscles and the smooth muscles in the gut.

In contrast to what people generally believe, muscles need energy to relax, not to contract. What happens on the electrocardiogram, or ECG, when part of the heart lacks oxygen illustrates this point. An electrocardiogram is a graph of the electrical activity of the heart when the different parts of it contract and relax.

The first part of the graph represents the electrical activity from contraction of the upper and lower chambers of the heart and the second part that from relaxation of the lower chambers. When lack of oxygen occurs, compromising energy metabolism, we see the resulting changes not in the first and contraction part of the electrocardiogram but in the second part, when the lower chambers relax.

In addition, the more active the muscles, the more the lack of metabolic energy affects their functioning. We divide the skeletal muscles in our body into postural muscles and movement muscles. The postural muscles maintain our erect posture and comprise the neck, shoulder, and upper back muscles, the lower back muscles, and the calf muscles. The jaw muscles are part of the postural muscle system as well, to keep our mouth closed when we are erect.

The postural muscles are the first to become tight when the body copes with a lack of metabolic energy, because they work the hardest to maintain our erect posture. When muscles are tight, they interfere with their blood supply, creating a vicious cycle that further deprives them of metabolic energy, causing more muscle tightness over time.

The interference with blood supply also causes the waste products that the blood ordinarily washes out of the muscles to accumulate. These waste products are acid, and the acidification of the tight muscles renders them sore and tender due to irritation of the pain nerve fibers that run through them. This, in turn, creates a vicious cycle of its own, resulting in yet more muscle tightness over time.

As you can see, these unfortunate postural muscles end up finding themselves in a very poor situation; it is, therefore, not surprising that they give us as much trouble as they do.

Poor Peristalsis

The smooth muscles in our gut wind up in a similarly dire situation, which may be less evident, but when it manifests itself, it does not give us any less misery.

Poor relaxation of the smooth muscles of the gut results in poor forward propulsion, or peristalsis, of stomach and large bowel content. As a result, the stomach and the large bowel fail to empty out well of acid and stool respectively.

When the stomach does not empty out its acid well, the acid ends up irritating its lining and causing gastritis, resulting in complaints like heartburn, reflux, nausea, or stomach pain. Tiny ulcers lead to blood loss, which over time causes iron deficiency and low hemoglobin, or anemia, both important and treatable causes of fatigue.

The poor emptying out of the stool by the large bowel causes it to harden due to the extraction of water, which is one of the functions of the large bowel. It renders the stool difficult to evacuate, and constipation develops with infrequent bowel movements and hard stool. The evacuation then becomes incomplete and unsatisfactory and may be painful, creating another vicious cycle.

The associated straining is a cause of hemorrhoids, which may bleed with every bowel movement, also potentially causing blood loss over time. The hard stool itself can cause tears in the lining of the anus, referred to as fissures, which are not only very painful but can bleed as well.

The constipation is sometimes accompanied by abdominal discomfort or pain, usually cramping that happens before a bowel movement is due and relieved afterward. When this is the case, we refer to the condition as constipation-predominant irritable bowel syndrome, or IBS-C.

The constipation can result in diarrhea, known as paradoxical diarrhea, which is really the body's effort to try to pass the hard stool. The diarrhea builds up behind it, usually at the cost of severe pain due to distension of the bowel.

The distension of the bowel causes cramps that are supposed to move the hard stool forward, if possible to the point of evacuation. However, sometimes the diarrhea just passes by it, causing significant suffering without gain. Under those circumstances, it is important to inspect the stool to ascertain that the diarrhea does, indeed, evacuate at least some of the hard stool.

When the above is the case, it is important to realize that constipation is the problem even though the diarrhea may be the most bothersome complaint, and that the treatment is with stool softeners, laxatives, or both. The paradoxical diarrhea changes the constipation-predominant irritable bowel syndrome, or IBS-C, into what we call mixed irritable bowel syndrome, or IBS-M.

Constipation alternating with diarrhea is the most typical presentation of irritable bowel syndrome. Usually, there is no bowel movement for a couple of days, followed by gradually increasing lower abdominal distension, or bloating, and pain, culminating in explosive diarrhea. Again, the treatment is with stool softeners, laxatives, or both and not with antidiarrheal medications, such as loperamide, which make the situation worse.

Lack of Sleep

We often do not realize that tightness of muscles, especially in the neck, shoulders, and upper back, as invariably present in chronic migraineurs, can be a significant cause of insomnia. It may not be those muscles in particular, however, but in order to fall asleep, we need to relax not only our mind but also our body, which means the muscles in our body.

When muscles are chronically tight, relaxation is difficult, and muscle tightness may well be the single most common cause of primary insomnia. With this kind of insomnia, the patient has problems falling asleep, sleeping through the night, and waking up early. Interrupted sleep is particularly detrimental to producing enough metabolic energy to last the day, but also, the total sleep time is important.

People with primary insomnia may not get more than four to six hours of sleep per night, which is by far not enough apart from its interrupted nature. Here, another vicious cycle presents itself with tight muscles that make relaxation problematic and, consequently, render it difficult to sleep. The lack of sleep causes a further shortage of metabolic energy, which, in turn, makes it even more onerous for the muscles to relax.

Of course, other problems can cause insomnia as well, such as a mind with racing thoughts that are difficult to quiet down, discomfort or pain, rendering it difficult to get comfortable in bed, restlessness of the legs with an irresistible urge to move them, or delayed sleep phase disorder. The latter is like living in a continuous state of jet lag.

Whatever the cause of the insomnia, however, it is paramount to remember that lack of sleep is the foremost cause of fatigue, also keeping in mind that it can be lifestyle related due to retiring too late at night, rising too early in the morning, or both.

Hormones

Menstrual cycle disorders, such as infrequent menstruation, frequent menstruation, or irregular menstrual cycle, and menstruation disorders, like heavy, long, or painful menstruation, both comorbid with chronic migraine in particular, suggest that there is hormonal, or endocrine, involvement as well.

This hormonal involvement may align with the chronic fatigue if there is a thyroid component to its cause, fully or in part. The hormonal systems in the body act in close relation to each other, and a deranged function in one, however so slight, may set off that of others.

I know from clinical experience that the menstrual cycle and menstruation are very sensitive to changes in thyroid function. Prescribing patients even a small amount of the thyroid hormone levothyroxine, such as twenty-five or fifty micrograms per day, may immediately straighten out any irregularities in menstrual cycle or menstruation, also when the thyroid function is within the laboratory's reference range.

Such menstrual cycle or menstruation irregularities are commonly associated with infertility, which I have seen resolved as well with a small dose of levothyroxine, even in somewhat older women. As a result, I have become very vigilant about abnormal thyroid function when menstrual cycle or menstruation disorders are comorbid with migraine.

They can occur with too high or too low thyroid function, which means with overactive as well as with underactive thyroid. However, I have encountered them much more frequently with low thyroid function, or hypothyroidism, than with high thyroid function, or hyperthyroidism, probably because the former is up to five times more common than the latter.

Both can cause fatigue, and one can go into the other, or they can alternate, especially in a disorder known as Hashimoto's thyroiditis. In this condition, the body forms antibodies against the thyroid gland, such as thyroid peroxidase antibody, or TPO-a, and thyroglobulin antibody, or TG-a.

These antibodies inflame the thyroid gland, causing thyroiditis, and over time destroy it, with active inflammation associated with hyperthyroidism and the destruction over time resulting in hypothyroidism. The elevated level of thyroid peroxidase antibody may also itself in part be causative of the fatigue characteristic of the disorder.

Psychiatric Comorbidities

How exactly the psychiatric comorbidities of migraine—that is, anxiety and depression—fit into the picture is more difficult to explain and probably even more complicated. Anxiety and depression are related conditions, and both are comorbid with migraine regardless of the presentation, but much more so with chronic migraine than with episodic migraine.

Studies suggest that anxiety, if present, precedes the onset of migraine while depression follows it, but such a linear causal relation, although plausible, seems too simple an explanation. Anxiety and depression, on the one hand, and migraine, on the other, are succinctly different disorders. Depression may very well develop out of anxiety, anxiety may make migraine worse, and migraine may aggravate depression; anything beyond that is unlikely, in my opinion.

Apart from the fact that they may make each other worse in a bidirectional manner—and in most cases, they probably do—anxiety and depression are conditions separate from migraine, not linked by underlying mechanism.

Systemic Syndrome

I believe that the linked comorbidities, as explained, share a lack of metabolic energy, manifesting itself in fatigue, as their underlying mechanism. This problem with energy metabolism is systemic, involving the body as a whole, and undoubtedly has a hormonal component as well. For these reasons, I refer to it as systemic endocrine-metabolic syndrome, or SEMS.

The syndrome encompasses the multitude of disorders that I have explained throughout as caused by a lack of metabolic energy. This means that the people afflicted by it, in actuality, have one condition rather than several, and that they are not crazy or hypochondriacs. They have a disorder that affects something very fundamental to life, which is the energy supply to the cells in their body. Headache is part of that syndrome, but migraine explicitly is not, as illustrated by the following patient vignette.

A thirty-four-year-old woman has developed pressure in her temples, tightness in her jaws, and pain in her shoulders following pregnancy. Apart from these complaints, she has long and heavy periods, lasting eight or nine days, which were very painful from menarche until the pregnancy. The periods occur regularly and on a monthly basis, but she has infertility issues nevertheless.

Her stomach area is tender, and she has constipation-predominant irritable bowel syndrome. She also has anxiety. She sleeps well and gets seven or eight hours of sleep per night, but she feels tired during the day nevertheless and weak in general.

Migraine appears in the picture when the genetically determined and inherited vulnerability for that condition is present as well. Its presentation under those circumstances is that of chronic migraine because of the chronic tightness of the neck, shoulder, upper back, and jaw muscles associated with the syndrome. This explains why particularly chronic migraine and not episodic migraine is associated with the comorbidities attributed above to a lack of metabolic energy.

As explained, I do not believe that the psychiatric comorbidities, anxiety and depression, are part of the systemic endocrine-metabolic syndrome. They are definitely more commonly associated with chronic migraine than with episodic migraine, because chronic migraine is worse and, probably, also because of the multiple comorbid disorders associated with it. This undoubtedly makes life even more onerous to bear for the chronic migraineur than it already is and makes it much more difficult to cope with the headaches, which is often already a problem when they occur episodically.

Chapter 11

Which Medications Prevent Migraine?

Migraine Prevention

The preventive treatment of migraine headaches with medications—in other words, pharmacological migraine prevention—comes in three forms: long-term prevention, short-term prevention, and prevention of the last chance or preemptive prevention. Of these, long-term prevention is the best known. It has the most medications available, and we prescribe them the most, but unfortunately, not often enough. As a result, numerous migraineurs continue to suffer unnecessarily.

It involves the ongoing use of medication administered daily, every other day, monthly, or quarterly to prevent the occurrence of headaches over time. The frequency of medication intake is determined by its duration of action, which in turn, depends on how long it stays in the body. Regular medications stay in the body for hours or days, and so-called biologics, like antibodies, last for weeks, if not months.

Short-term migraine prevention aims at averting migraine headaches at times of increased vulnerability, such as around menstruation—that is, perimenstrually—or on weekends. We can apply it as well when migraine headaches are particularly undesirable, such as at a wedding or graduation. Then the patient takes the medication for a short period, ranging from a couple of days to a week or so.

Evidence exists for several triptans to prevent menstrual migraine headaches when taken daily for five to seven days perimenstrually, starting two days before the expected menstruation. These are frovatriptan, naratriptan, and zolmitriptan—all in dosages of 2.5 milligrams twice daily. The first two are longer-acting triptans, but that does not seem to matter because zolmitriptan does the same, although lasting much shorter.

Therefore, any triptan can be used, if necessary, for short-term migraine prevention, not only to prevent headaches perimenstrually but also, for example, to ascertain that they do not spoil weekends or special occasions. I have employed the same strategy with unrelenting migraine headaches, having the patient take a triptan on a regular schedule twice daily for two days, followed by half the dose twice daily for two days.

Prevention of the last chance or preemptive prevention is the least well-known and, consequently, rarely utilized. It also has the fewest treatment options and is the most difficult to apply. The patient takes the medication to prevent a migraine headache that is imminent, based on an assessment of premonitory complaints, or prodromes. It requires the consistent occurrence of those symptoms before the onset of the headache by hours, which makes it predictable with a relatively high degree of certainty. Otherwise, it will only result in the random intake of medication with little or no benefit.

There is evidence for effective preemptive treatment of migraine headaches with the anti-nausea and gastrokinetic medication domperidone in the dose of thirty milligrams and with the gepant ubrogepant in the dose of one hundred milligrams. I have similar experience with another anti-nausea and gastrokinetic medication metoclopramide in the dose of ten milligrams, taken during the migraine aura and preventing the subsequent headache.

Both anti-nausea and gastrokinetic medications block the receptor of a chemical in the body called dopamine, with the difference that metoclopramide enters the brain while domperidone does not. The gepants also do not penetrate the brain, and neither do the triptans, which all may well have similar benefit, although we never studied them in this way.

Adjunct Treatment

We should never use preventive migraine treatment, pharmacological or non-pharmacological, on its own regardless of what it consists of. We should always apply it as adjunct treatment added to effective abortive treatment, which I consider the foundation of long-term migraine management. Without it, long-term migraine prevention is an illusion, with each suffered migraine headache setting the patient back.

I only consider abortive migraine treatment effective if it *fully* relieves the headaches within two hours and does so consistently and without side effects. Anything other than that, as far as I am concerned, needs further work. In the vast majority of patients, we can accomplish effective abortive treatment as defined, although it may take some time and effort.

Whether an indication exists for adding preventive treatment is a matter of discussion between the patient and the physician or other health care practitioner. There are criteria for prescribing preventive migraine treatment in terms of the number of headache days per month. Of course, these are arbitrary and do not take the particular situation of the patient into account. With migraine headaches that happen on a monthly basis, we should consider preventive treatment, and we should think about it harder the more often they occur and the longer they last.

With effective abortive treatment, most migraine headaches can be limited in duration to one or two hours. However, particularly with headaches that happen in relation to the menstrual cycle, treatment may be required for several consecutive days. Depending on the lifestyle, this may be hard to manage, or it may be a sufficient source of stress to make life more difficult, generating anxiety and, consequently, more headaches.

Think about it if you do not have migraine or if you belong to the fortunate group of migraineurs with occasional headaches only. Having to deal with something regularly that disables you for the day or, if not that bad, interferes with your ability to function can be quite stressful and anxiety provoking.

Anxiety is a well-known trigger of headaches, including migraine headaches, and regularly occurring headaches generate it, especially when severe and disabling. Therefore, with migraine headaches that happen regularly, and after establishing effective abortive treatment, it is important to discuss preventive treatment and review the available options.

Comorbidities

Effective long-term migraine prevention is equally an illusion in the presence of active comorbidities that make the patient feel miserable overall. Headaches are sensitive to whatever goes on internally, physically or mentally, and externally.

Anxiety drives headache frequency, and depression makes it more difficult to cope with them. Fatigue is probably the biological reason we experience headaches, and insomnia is a common cause of fatigue. Both are especially a problem when persistent and are important to consider and, if possible, to treat. It is also paramount to examine for potential medical causes of fatigue, which would generally require the performance of blood tests.

If insomnia is present and not due to lifestyle, it is important to look at possible causes, such as racing thoughts preventing falling asleep or physical discomfort or pain making sleeping in general difficult. It is paramount to consider other conditions as explanations of insomnia as well, such as restless legs syndrome, or RLS, and delayed sleep phase disorder.

Musculoskeletal disorders are often the cause of physical discomfort or pain, potentially affecting daily functioning and sleep. They are common comorbidities of migraine, especially of its chronic variant, in which chronic tightness of the neck, shoulder, and upper back muscles is invariably present. Often present as well are chronic tightness of the jaw muscles, causing temporomandibular disorder, or TMD; chronic tightness of the low back muscles, causing chronic low back pain, or lumbago; and chronic tightness of the calf muscles, causing nocturnal cramps or charley horses in the lower legs or feet.

The chronic muscle tightness is, in my opinion, not from stress but from the comorbid chronic fatigue, indicating a lack of metabolic energy that impairs muscle relaxation. Impaired muscle relaxation also makes the forward movement of the stomach-bowel system, referred to as gastrointestinal peristalsis, slow, resulting in gastritis and large bowel problems, such as chronic constipation and irritable bowel syndrome, or IBS.

These conditions not only render life more difficult and miserable but also potentially cause headaches. In addition, they make it more arduous for the migraineur to tolerate the headaches and cope with them mentally and physically.

Ideally, we add a preventive migraine medication when we have met the following prerequisites.

First, the patient is receiving effective abortive migraine treatment that relieves the headaches *fully* within two hours and does so consistently and without side effects.

Second, we have treated any comorbid disorder present to the extent possible, which is especially important in the patient with chronic migraine.

Third, the patient adheres to general lifestyle measures, such as eating regularly and not skipping meals, getting enough sleep by going to bed on time and not oversleeping in the morning, avoiding excessive consumption of caffeine and alcohol, and spreading activities over the day while regularly taking a break to avoid excessive fatigue.

Fourth, effective dialogue between the patient and the physician or other health care practitioner ensures compliance with the preventive treatment, which requires daily, every other day, monthly, or quarterly administration of medication, potentially for an extended period.

Medications

The medications that are available for preventive migraine treatment with demonstrated efficacy, tolerability, and safety in multiple clinical trials I divide into two categories: old-fashioned and standard-of-care.

The former are not specific to migraine, and we did not advance them specifically for migraine treatment, whether abortive or preventive. We developed them for the treatment of other conditions, such as depression (tricyclics, 1950s), high blood pressure and angina of the heart (beta-blockers, 1960s; calcium antagonists, 1970s), and epilepsy (anticonvulsants, 1930s). The discovery of their benefit in migraine was serendipity.

As far as I am concerned, we should no longer prescribe them in favor of those specifically advanced for the preventive treatment of migraine, which are also much more effective. The development of medications in general has changed significantly over the last several decades, with much more emphasis on tolerability and safety. The more recently advanced ones are safer, especially with long-term use, and are better tolerated with fewer, if any, side effects.

We can add to that the development of antibodies as medications, which in my opinion constitute the future of medicine. They are highly targeted with little, if any, so-called off-target activity, generally conveying great tolerability and safety. Their long duration of action, often covering months, requires infrequent administration and, thus, assures better compliance.

The two classes of medications that we specifically advanced for migraine prevention are the CGRP antibodies, also referred to as CGRP monoclonal antibodies, or mAbs, and the small molecule CGRP receptor antagonists, or gepants. Both classes target the CGRP pathway, as we call it, with the acronym standing for calcitonin gene-related peptide.

Serotonin Antagonists

We often forget that there is yet another class of medications, specifically developed for the preventive treatment of migraine. This is the class of the so-called serotonin antagonists that includes methysergide and its successor, pizotifen. Sandoz Laboratories in Basel, Switzerland, advanced the former in the 1960s based on a theory proposed by the Italian master of migraine, Federigo Sicuteri.

Professor Sicuteri was an internist and clinical pharmacologist interested in inflammation as it relates to pain, especially the pain of migraine. His interest focused on the chemicals in the body that potentially cause pain, such as bradykinin and serotonin. He found that migraineurs, when studied during migraine headaches, excreted an increased amount of a breakdown product of serotonin in their urine. He consequently suggested that a serotonin storm causes the migraine headache, with the platelets in the blood being the source of the released serotonin.

In order to counteract the impact of the serotonin storm, Sandoz developed methysergide as a potent serotonin antagonist from the psychedelic drug lysergic acid diethylamide, or LSD. It proved very effective as a preventive migraine medication, but its efficacy came with a significant downside, involving scarring of the heart, lungs, and kidneys. The company subsequently advanced pizotifen, but it was by far not as effective, probably because, unlike methysergide, it is not an ergot.

As an ergot, methysergide has enough vasoconstrictor activity to increase the tone of the blood vessels in the head. By doing so, it hampers their widening that occurs as part of the migraine headache mechanism. The beta-blockers prevent migraine headaches in a similar way by increasing blood vessel tone, although they are not vasoconstrictors.

The patient should take pizotifen once daily at bedtime, because it can cause drowsiness, starting with a dose of 0.5 milligram, which they can gradually increase, if necessary, to 3 milligrams. Apart from drowsiness, it can cause dry mouth and light-headedness, as well as increased appetite and weight gain. The latter side effects are probably due to the increase in blood insulin level that happens with prolonged use of the medication.

Pizotifen does not have contraindications, but we should avoid it in patients with increased eye pressure due to glaucoma or with complaints related to an enlarged prostate, such as difficulty urinating and frequent urination, especially at night, called nocturia.

Tricyclics

At least structurally, pizotifen is similar to the so-called tricyclics that we developed in the 1950s for the treatment of depression. Imipramine was the first one to come to market, in 1959, followed by amitriptyline, the best known in its class in 1961.

We studied amitriptyline initially in chronic tension headache, which is a low-grade headache that is present most or all the time, because we considered it a manifestation of depression. When it proved to be effective, we also investigated it in migraine and found it beneficial there as well.

We use amitriptyline for headache prevention in much lower dosages than for the treatment of depression, generally twenty-five to one hundred milligrams per day as opposed to two hundred to four hundred milligrams. It has a relatively long duration of action, which means that the patient takes it just once daily, preferably at bedtime, because it causes drowsiness.

Apart from drowsiness, it can cause dry mouth and constipation; more importantly, however, it stimulates appetite and brings about weight gain. The latter side effects make me reluctant to prescribe it to women in particular, because they often already struggle with their weight. In addition, patients with increased eye pressure due to glaucoma, enlarged prostate, epilepsy, or heart disease should avoid it as well.

If I use amitriptyline for chronic tension headache or migraine prevention, I start with a small dose, sometimes as low as 10 or 12.5 milligrams, once daily at bedtime. I subsequently very gradually increase it until the patient experiences some dryness of the mouth. I do not want the mouth to be cotton dry, but some dryness indicates that the medication is in the body at a therapeutic level.

As I very gradually increase the dose, I monitor the patient carefully for fatigue as a side effect in an attempt not to cause it or make it worse. Fatigue is a common trigger of headaches, including migraine headaches, and causing or worsening it with a preventive medication negates its potential benefit.

If I consider there to be an indication for a tricyclic, which is generally the case in chronic tension headache but no longer in migraine, I prefer imipramine to amitriptyline because patients tolerate it better with less side effects. I prescribe it in similar dosages to amitriptyline.

Sometimes, we use doxepin instead of amitriptyline, also in similar dosages, but it potentially causes the same side effects—namely, drowsiness, dry mouth, constipation, stimulation of appetite, and weight gain.

An alternative to imipramine that I may employ is nortriptyline, also prescribed in similar dosages, which patients tolerate equally well. However, the evidence for the effectiveness of either tricyclic in chronic tension headache is limited, if present at all.

Beta-Blockers

The next class of preventive migraine medications is that of the so-called beta-blockers. We originally developed them for the treatment of high blood pressure, or hypertension, and angina of the heart, also called angina pectoris. Narrowing of blood vessels of the heart underlies the latter condition and causes the chest pain on physical exertion, sometimes radiating into the left arm or jaw, characteristic of it.

The first medication advanced in this class was propranolol, which became available in 1967. We discovered its beneficial effect in migraine prevention by chance, or serendipitously, while studying it in patients with angina of the heart who also had migraine.

We have good evidence for the effectiveness of six beta-blockers in migraine prevention, which are, in alphabetical order, atenolol, bisoprolol, metoprolol, nadolol, propranolol, and timolol. They share the particular feature of increasing blood vessel tone, which prevents the blood vessels in the head from widening as much as they would otherwise. Their dosages for the preventive treatment of migraine are similar to those that we use for the treatment of hypertension or angina pectoris.

The most commonly prescribed beta-blocker for migraine prevention is propranolol, which I never use, because it has the most side effects. I think that the underlying reason is that apart from its effect on the blood vessels that is beneficial to migraine headaches, it also decreases thyroid function. It does so by inhibiting the activation of the thyroid prohormone levothyroxine, or T4, to the thyroid hormone triiodothyronine, or T3.

A good working thyroid gland should be able to compensate for this effect of the medication, but my concern is that many people, unfortunately, do not have a thyroid that works sufficiently well.

Fatigue is the most frequent side effect of beta-blockers in general, which is an important issue in migraine prevention, because it is a common cause of headaches, including migraine headaches. Therefore, if I use a beta-blocker for migraine prevention, which I still sometimes do, I always start with a low dose—for example, 25 milligrams of atenolol per day, 2.5 milligrams of bisoprolol per day, 25 milligrams of metoprolol per day, 20 milligrams of nadolol per day, or 2.5 milligrams of timolol per day.

Here also, I very gradually increase the dose, taking my time, until the patient has a heart rate of fifty to sixty beats per minute, indicating that the beta-blocker is in the body at a therapeutic level. While I do this, I track the patient's blood pressure as well, because after all, these medications treat hypertension by lowering blood pressure. More importantly, however, I monitor the occurrence or worsening of fatigue, which may negate the medication's migraine preventive benefit.

I think that ensuing fatigue is also often the reason why the benefit of beta-blockers in preventing migraine headaches wears off over time. If this happens, I address it by lowering the dose of the medication, often with return of the headache preventive benefit once the fatigue has improved.

Apart from fatigue, propranolol in particular causes depression, insomnia, and impotence. Patients with low blood pressure, or hypotension; low heart rate, or bradycardia; or lung disease, including asthma, should avoid beta-blockers for migraine prevention or for any other indication.

Calcium Antagonists

Another class of preventive migraine medications initially developed for the treatment of hypertension and angina of the heart, or angina pectoris, is that of the calcium channel blockers or calcium entry blockers, also referred to as calcium antagonists. We advanced them in the 1960s and 1970s, and verapamil was the first one to come to market, which was in 1981. Shortly after it became available, we showed it to be beneficial in migraine prevention, and several others followed suit, with nimodipine having the best evidence of benefit.

In the United States, we mostly prescribe verapamil as a calcium antagonist for migraine prevention, generally in dosages of 80 or 120 milligrams three times per day. Its most common side effect is constipation, and we should avoid it in patients with electrical conduction issues of the heart.

In Europe, a commonly used calcium antagonist for migraine prevention is flunarizine, which we specifically developed for that purpose. The dose is ten milligrams taken once daily at bedtime, because it can cause drowsiness; it sometimes also causes weight gain. Flunarizine does not have contraindications for its use.

Anticonvulsants

The last class of medications not specifically advanced for the preventive treatment of migraine but found by chance, or serendipitously, to be helpful is that of the anti-seizure medications, or anticonvulsants. This class has been around for over a century and a half, and we have used them for the treatment of chronic pain for eighty years.

For migraine prevention, we studied two anticonvulsants in particular—namely, topiramate and valproate—which got official approval for the migraine indication in 2004 and 2008 respectively. Apart from the fact that they are not specific to migraine, the problem with both medications is that patients do not tolerate them well because of side effects.

Common side effects of topiramate are fatigue and drowsiness, as well as tingling of the hands or feet. However and much more important, it can impair memory, especially word retrieval, and thinking, or cognition, the latter sometimes not recognized until the patient discontinues it—for example, due to lack of benefit. Common side effects of valproate are fatigue, drowsiness, indigestion, nausea, diarrhea, and weight gain.

I no longer prescribe either medication because of the generally poor tolerability. Especially if cognitive side effects occur, they negatively affect the patient's ability to function at home, as well as at work or at school. The dose of topiramate is 25 or 50 milligrams once or twice daily, and that of valproate is 250 or 500 milligrams twice daily. We should avoid the latter in patients with abnormal liver function.

Old-Fashioned

Apart from imipramine or nortriptyline, which I may still use occasionally for the treatment of chronic tension headache, or a beta-blocker with the exception of propranolol for migraine prevention, I no longer prescribe the aforementioned nonspecific preventive migraine medications. I consider them old-fashioned and cannot emphasize enough that the current standard of care relies on specific medications, whether it is for the treatment of migraine or for that of any of its comorbid conditions.

The specific medications for the abortive treatment of migraine are the triptans and the gepants, and for migraine prevention, they are the CGRP antibodies and the gepants. Specifically for the preventive treatment of chronic migraine, botulinum toxin still has a role to play but, in my opinion, a diminished one. The CGRP antibodies and gepants are much easier to administer and, at least in my experience, much more effective. In general, they provide a higher level of benefit that may commence within a week of treatment and, in addition, is much more stable over time.

In contrast, it easily takes ten to fourteen days for the botulinum toxin to provide relief, and it often already wears off two to three weeks before the next set of injections is due. Additionally, receiving thirty-one injections in the head, back of the neck, and shoulders is not a great experience, to say the least.

CGRP Antibodies

The four CGRP antibodies, also called CGRP monoclonal antibodies or mAbs are, in alphabetical order, eptinezumab, erenumab, fremanezumab, and galcanezumab. The acronym CGRP stands for *calcitonin gene-related peptide*, a peptide, or protein, in the body that potently widens blood vessels.

We did the so-called proof of concept study of the antibodies in migraine prevention with galcanezumab in 2012, and six years later, in 2018, three of them became available on the market. This is a remarkably short trajectory for the approval of medications, which typically takes a decade or longer and sometimes much longer. This short approval time is testimony to the great efficacy, tolerability, and safety of this class of preventive migraine medications.

As the medications are proteins, or peptides, we cannot take them by mouth, because the stomach digests them. Instead, we administer them parenterally, as we call it—erenumab, fremanezumab, and galcanezumab by injection under the skin, or subcutaneously, and eptinezumab by intravenous infusion.

Antibodies stay in the body for long periods, generally approximately one hundred days, but the CGRP antibodies remain in the body even longer—namely, five to six months. This means that we can administer them infrequently—that is, monthly or quarterly. For most patients, this is much easier than taking a medication daily, which is the case with those that we traditionally prescribe for the preventive treatment of migraine.

Compliance is better with infrequent administration, and this translates into potentially better benefit, because missing or late dosing is much less an issue. I think that this is what the future of medicine looks like: infrequent administration of long-acting medications and for migraine prevention, the future is here!

The gepants for migraine prevention, on the other hand, are tablets that patients take daily or every other day, much like the traditional preventive migraine medications. The every-other-day dosing in particular may be a challenge for patients to remember, and here I suggest taking the medication on fixed days of the week—namely, Monday, Wednesday, and Friday.

The three antibodies that we administer under the skin, or subcutaneously—erenumab, fremanezumab, and galcanezumab—come in auto-injectors for easy self-administration by the patient. In principle, they can perform the injections in the upper arm—that is, in the so-called deltoid area—in the thigh, or in the abdomen.

I strongly recommend that patients perform the injections into the skin of the abdomen. There is much more subcutaneous tissue, or fat, underneath the abdominal skin than in the upper arm or thigh. It is also much easier to see what you are doing when injecting into the abdominal skin, as opposed to when you perform the injections into the skin of the upper arm.

It is also easy to see when you inject into the skin of the thigh, but generally, the subcutaneous fat there is rather thin. Although the needles in the auto-injector devices are no longer than 0.4 inches, or 1 centimeter, injecting into the skin of the thigh easily ends up injecting into the underlying fascia.

The fascia is the connective tissue layer between the subcutaneous fat and the muscle—in this case, the quadriceps muscle. Injecting into it is painful, which a subcutaneous injection should hardly be, if at all. In addition, the absorption out of the fascia is poor, potentially resulting in reduced medication exposure and, hence, less benefit.

With subcutaneous injection of proteins like the CGRP antibodies, absorption into the blood is an issue, because the antibodies are too large to pass directly into the capillaries. This is not a problem with small-molecule medications given subcutaneously, such as, for example, the sumatriptan injection for abortive migraine treatment.

A small molecule like sumatriptan passes directly from the subcutaneous fat via the capillaries into the blood, which rapidly distributes it through the body. This is not the case with the antibodies administered subcutaneously, which the so-called lymphatic system takes up and carries to the blood.

This indirect passage via the lymphatic system to the blood creates a loss, which can be as high as 25–40 percent. Loss of antibody means less exposure and, consequently, less benefit. The problem is that we never know how much loss there is, and with no or inadequate improvement, this is a question we cannot answer.

Answering this question is possible only when we give the antibody by intravenous infusion, which brings it directly into the blood. This is feasible with the CGRP antibody called eptinezumab, which is available for intravenous administration only. There may be an advantage to initiating CGRP antibody treatment with eptinezumab given intravenously, securing 100 percent availability of the medication to prevent migraine headaches.

The standard dose is one hundred milligrams, which we infuse over a half hour every three months, or quarterly. Some medical offices have infusion capabilities, but this is a service certainly offered by most hospitals. In addition, home infusion resources are available as well, with a nurse coming to the house with the appropriate equipment and the medication.

Tolerability

The CGRP antibodies are either human or humanized, that is, mostly human, which makes the likelihood of an allergic reaction following their administration very low. However, a serious allergic reaction can happen, such as angioedema or anaphylaxis.

Angioedema is a swelling similar to hives but under the skin instead of on the surface, usually affecting the eyes and lips. It can also occur in the hands, feet, and throat, in the latter case potentially causing difficulty breathing.

Anaphylaxis is a very rare allergic reaction, associated with dangerously low blood pressure, which can be fatal if not addressed immediately. We treat both with epinephrine given by intramuscular injection, which is also available as an auto-injector for easy self-administration by the patient.

Overall, however, patients tolerate the CGRP antibodies very well, and the vast majority do not experience any side effects. Occasionally, we see a skin reaction with the subcutaneously administered antibodies—erenumab, fremanezumab, or galcanezumab. It generally consists of slightly elevated redness at the site of the injection due to inflammation, which can be itchy. We should not interpret the itchiness as indicating an allergic reaction, in which case the skin reaction looks different—namely, like urticaria or hives.

If the inflammation of the skin at the injection site causes soreness or pain, the patient can take a nonsteroidal anti-inflammatory pain medication, or analgesic, as needed, like ibuprofen or naproxen sodium. If the skin reaction is allergic and urticarial in nature, they can use an antihistamine, like diphenhydramine.

In neither case is there a need to discontinue the medication, nor have I generally seen the skin reaction to worsen over time with repeat administration. If the reaction is urticarial in nature, taking an antihistamine a half hour or so before the injection may mitigate it or prevent it altogether.

Constipation

With erenumab, constipation may ensue, which seems to be a potential side effect of medications that block the CGRP receptor. Apart from this medication, the gepants, which are small molecule CGRP receptor antagonists, block the CGRP receptor, potentially causing constipation as well. For them, however, this is relevant only when the patient takes the gepant daily and, hence, if there is enough exposure. This is not the case with intermittent intake—that is, when they use it as needed for abortive treatment or every other day preventively.

If constipation does happen with erenumab or with the daily use of a gepant, it is usually mild and easily treated with a stool softener, like docusate. I am much more concerned about it as a potential side effect in patients already constipated or who have irritable bowel syndrome, or IBS. Regarding the latter, this concern relates to the constipation-predominant and mixed presentations of the condition, IBS-C and IBS-M.

From a theoretical perspective, straight chronic diarrhea or diarrhea-predominant irritable bowel syndrome, or IBS-D, may improve with medications that block the CGRP receptor. However, I do not have the experience to state this for a fact, but I would not be surprised if those patients will enjoy some improvement of their bowel disorder.

Regarding irritable bowel syndrome, we should use CGRP receptor-blocking medications solely when there is diarrhea only, because if mixed with constipation or with not having a bowel movement for days and then having diarrhea, it will likely worsen.

The reason is that the mixed variety of irritable bowel syndrome, which is also its most typical presentation, is constipation-predominant irritable bowel syndrome gone awry. The diarrhea that occurs is paradoxical, because it happens as a result of the constipation; we should treat it as such with a stool softener, laxative, or both and never with an antidiarrheal medication, like loperamide.

If you have migraine and chronic constipation or irritable bowel syndrome, especially if the latter is of the constipation or mixed variety, it is important that we treat them as part of the long-term management of the headaches. If the irritable bowel syndrome is of the diarrhea type, we should treat it as well, but more because of its social than medical consequences, which also applies to chronic diarrhea.

My experience is that these conditions are especially distressing because of the need to be close to a restroom at all times. As the diarrhea is worse in the morning, those afflicted may not be able to leave home in a timely fashion to go to work or to school, experiencing considerable stress as a result. Of course, with diarrhea-predominant irritable bowel syndrome, significant discomfort or pain accompanies the diarrhea, which is of medical significance as well in relation to the comorbid migraine.

With either disorder—that is, chronic diarrhea or diarrhea-predominant irritable bowel syndrome—we should not rely on medications taken as-needed, such as the aforementioned antidiarrheal loperamide. As is also the case with constipation, we should take medication daily to regulate the bowel movements long-term, aiming at one or two bowel movements per day.

I have positive experience with a medication that we used to prescribe for migraine prevention—namely, amitriptyline—for the treatment of chronic diarrhea and diarrhea-predominant irritable bowel syndrome. I have seen it beneficial in those conditions in dosages even lower than we were accustomed prescribing for the prevention of migraine headaches. A dose as low as five or ten milligrams per day may treat both the diarrhea and the abdominal discomfort or pain that accompanies it in diarrhea-predominant irritable bowel syndrome.

If such a low dose does not provide the desired benefit, I suggest that, like in migraine treatment, we gradually increase it until there is some dryness of the mouth. It indicates that the medication is in the body in the amount necessary to have a so-called anticholinergic effect, which is what slows down large bowel activity.

Amitriptyline influences the serotonin system as well, which is what we think makes it valuable in the treatment of chronic pain. If increased appetite or weight gain is a concern, as they often were when we prescribed it for migraine prevention, we should employ another tricyclic, such as imipramine or nortriptyline.

The best way to treat chronic constipation or constipation-predominant or mixed irritable bowel syndrome, IBS-C or IBS-M, is with a daily regimen of a stool softener and, if necessary, with a laxative. The goal of the treatment is daily or near-daily bowel movements with stool of normal or near-normal consistency and not requiring excessive straining.

The two stool softeners that I use for this purpose are docusate in one-hundred-milligram capsules and magnesium citrate in two-hundred-milligram tablets. Both are not really medications, because they do not get absorbed into the body. They stay in the large bowel and prevent it from extracting excess fluid from the stool, which would otherwise make it hard and difficult to evacuate.

In my experience, magnesium citrate is more potent than docusate; consequently, I generally start with the latter in a dose of

200 milligrams per day. Depending on the response, I increase it to 400 milligrams or add senna in a dose of two tablets at bedtime, 8.6 milligrams each. I may further increase the dose or change it to magnesium citrate, usually in a dose of 400 milligrams per day.

If the stool consistency is better but the bowel movements are still infrequent, there is a need for an added laxative, like senna. If I can, however, I treat the chronic constipation or constipation-predominant or mixed irritable bowel syndrome with a stool softener only, even if it requires a relatively high dose of whatever I use.

As far as I am concerned, patients should not shy away from utilizing the aforementioned medications in dosages that provide the desired benefit. It does not make sense to take a medication for any disorder, whatever it is, in a dose that does not provide relief unless tolerability is an issue. Then it is obviously not the right one, and we should change it.

We have plenty of medications at our disposal and should make every effort to find the one that the patient tolerates well with no or minimal side effects. This, by the way, applies to the treatment of any condition, and we should consider it the standard of care. Excellent tolerability is what we can and should expect from any treatment, whatever it is.

Safety

Apart from the relatively small issues mentioned earlier, excellent tolerability is definitely a feature of the CGRP antibodies, whether given subcutaneously or intravenously. Their safety looks equally good, although we only have a little more than a decade experience with them, research and practice combined.

The antibodies block 90–95 percent of CGRP activity in the body, evidently without ill effects. Initially, we were concerned that calcitonin gene-related peptide, as a potent vasodilator, plays a role in blood pressure regulation. As a result, the first studies excluded patients with high blood pressure, or hypertension, from participation, even if it was well-controlled, and those taking antihypertensive medications for whatever reason. However, very quickly, it became evident that such restrictions were unnecessary because of a lack of effect of the antibodies on blood pressure.

Another concern is that lacking the availability of calcitonin gene-related peptide in the body would make a heart attack or brain attack—that is, a stroke—bigger if it happens under treatment with a CGRP antibody or gepant. Apart from the fact that this concern does not have much of a scientific foundation, it would take a long time to know, if we ever find out.

Over the last several decades, medicine has made tremendous progress preventing and treating cardiovascular and cerebrovascular disease. In addition, people between the ages of fifteen and forty-five carry the bulk of the migraine burden; in that age group, these disorders are very uncommon. Age is a risk factor for numerous conditions but not for migraine, which, if anything, improves as we get older, especially in women once they reach menopause.

Dosing

With regard to the subcutaneously administered CGRP antibodies that we inject under the skin, galcanezumab comes with a loading dose of 240 milligrams, consisting of two injections of 120 milligrams each. Its purpose is to ascertain that the medication is already in the body at its maximum level in the first month of treatment.

Without a loading dose, it takes three to four months to reach the maximum level in the body, and this applies as well to the other two subcutaneously administered CGRP antibodies, erenumab and fremanezumab. After the loading dose, we give the galcanezumab monthly in the standard dose of 120 milligrams.

We always administer erenumab in a dose of 70 milligrams monthly and fremanezumab in that of 225 milligrams monthly. With erenumab, we have the option of increasing the monthly dose from 70 milligrams to 140 milligrams; with fremanezumab, we have the option of administering it quarterly as opposed to monthly. With the quarterly dosing, we give three injections at a time for a total of 675 milligrams.

The quarterly administration may be particularly convenient for college students who do not want to take the auto-injectors to their dormitories or during the summer, avoiding the need to travel with them. The latter is important because we need to keep the auto-injectors refrigerated until use, to be taken out approximately thirty minutes beforehand to allow them to warm up to room temperature.

Despite the loading dose for galcanezumab, I advise patients to stay on a CGRP antibody for at least three or four months before making a final judgment as to its benefit. At that point, it is important to reflect on the efficacy of the medication, because as aforementioned, tolerability is hardly ever an issue.

Initially, I questioned patients separately about the frequency and intensity of their headaches to determine whether there is more benefit on one than on the other. Due to the way the CGRP antibodies work, I anticipated more impact on headache intensity than on headache frequency. There is obviously a connection between the two in the sense that when the intensity of headaches drops to zero, headache frequency, by definition, goes down.

Accordingly, patients generally related a benefit on both, and I have since inquired about the improvement in overall migraine condition only. I ask patients, if possible, to give me an overall assessment in terms of a percentage. Most are able to do so, although sometimes, I have to help them a little, considering the effect on headache frequency and headache intensity separately and then putting the two together in a single percentage.

Unique to the CGRP antibodies and gepants, it is quite common for patients to give me high numbers of improvement that are in the 80s or 90s, sometimes even 100 percent. As a result, I have come to expect an overall improvement in migraine headaches of minimally 50 percent, combining the effects on frequency and intensity.

If the patient gives me anything less than that, I will increase the dose from 100 to 300 milligrams when they are on eptinezumab and from 70 to 140 milligrams when they are on erenumab. With fremanezumab and galcanezumab, increasing the dose is not an option; therefore, I will switch to another one. In general, it is important, however, not to give up on a class of medications unless we have tried at least several members of it.

This is not only paramount for the CGRP antibodies, of which we have four, but also for the triptans, of which we have seven, the beta-blockers for migraine prevention, of which we have six, and the gepants, of which we have three for abortive treatment and two for preventive treatment.

It is certainly possible for a patient not to tolerate a particular medication out of a class or not respond to it while tolerating another one well or responding to it. This is also the case with the CGRP antibodies, and I recommend that patients, if necessary, try all four because of the potential benefit.

If tolerability is an issue, it is important to try to understand the side effect in terms of its underlying mechanism and proceed accordingly rather than randomly picking another medication, as I unfortunately see too often. For example, if constipation is an issue with any of the CGRP-targeted medications, whether antibody or gepant, the answer may be one that works on the CGRP molecule, or ligand, rather than on the CGRP receptor.

Regarding the triptans, nausea seems to be a specific side effect of sumatriptan, related to its mild slowing effect on gastric emptying. Fortunately, we have the option here of prescribing any other triptan instead. With a so-called triptan side effect, such as upper chest or throat tightness, it makes sense to switch to a slower-acting one, like frovatriptan or naratriptan.

With regard to the beta-blockers for migraine prevention, switching from propranolol to another one often improves tolerability dramatically because of its effect on thyroid function. In this context, it is important to remember that we uniquely prescribe it for the treatment of symptoms associated with overactive thyroid, or hyperthyroidism.

Gepants

Along with the CGRP antibodies, the gepants, or small molecule CGRP receptor antagonists, are medications specifically developed for the treatment of migraine. While we advanced the CGRP antibodies for migraine prevention, we developed the gepants for abortive *and* preventive treatment.

This does not mean, however, that the CGRP antibodies cannot work abortively, because we have shown this to be the case for the one administered intravenously—namely, eptinezumab. It would be great if emergency room physicians employed it instead of the cocktail of medications they give migraine patients when coming in for a severe headache.

The majority of them who visit emergency rooms every so often have frequent headaches and, hence, suffer from chronic migraine. Due to the high frequency of their headaches, they would significantly benefit from a medication like eptinezumab, which not only relieves the severe headache they seek treatment for but also effectively prevents them for months thereafter.

The subcutaneously administered CGRP antibodies do not offer this immediate benefit, but they can certainly provide preventive migraine headache relief within a week. When we use a gepant preventively, we can also see the benefit within a week, if not sooner, because they work abortively as well. We have two gepants that we can prescribe preventively, one of which, rimegepant, we can also employ for abortive treatment.

Rimegepant comes in one dose and in one formulation only, which is the seventy-five-milligram orally disintegrating tablet, or ODT. The patient takes one tablet for abortive migraine treatment, which they cannot repeat within twenty-four hours, or one tablet every other day for preventive treatment. If used preventively, I recommend that they do not take it every other day, because that is difficult to remember, but on Monday, Wednesday, and Friday instead for better compliance.

The other gepant for preventive migraine treatment, atogepant, the patient uses daily like the traditional preventive migraine medications; it comes in three dosages, which are ten, thirty, and sixty milligrams. I always advise patients to take it at bedtime rather than in the morning, because it can cause drowsiness, and of course, they can do the same with rimegepant when employed preventively.

Apart from drowsiness and when used abortively or preventively, gepants can cause fatigue, nausea, and constipation but do so in a very small percentage of patients only.

The sole safety concern with the gepants is the simultaneous use of a strong inhibitor of a liver enzyme system called CYP3A4. Important in this regard are the antiviral and antifungal medications, the former currently more relevant because of the COVID-19 pandemic. We can prescribe atogepant along with a strong CYP3A4 inhibitor, but just in its lowest dose of ten milligrams per day, which is also the one that we should use in patients with significant kidney disease.

As we can employ rimegepant abortively *and* preventively, probably a good way of prescribing it is for abortive treatment and for short-term prevention. The latter implies that the patient takes it preventively in the every-other-day dosing schedule for short periods and only when needed.

This can be around menstruation, or perimenstrually, if that is the time when the headaches are most likely to happen. Some migraineurs are especially vulnerable on weekends, so they could take it on Friday evening. They can also use it preventively when an important event is coming up, such as an exam, graduation, or wedding, they cannot miss.

From an episodic and chronic migraine perspective, the CGRP antibodies and atogepant are broad-spectrum preventive migraine medications, because they are effective in both. However, for atogepant in chronic migraine, we have demonstrated this to be the case solely for the sixty-milligram dose.

Like the old-fashioned preventive migraine medications, we have only shown benefit for rimegepant in episodic migraine; then we still have botulinum toxin, which has demonstrated efficacy limited to chronic migraine.

Botulinum Toxin

I do not consider botulinum toxin to be specific migraine treatment, because as far as I am concerned, it does not treat migraine; otherwise, it would be effective in episodic migraine as well. Instead, I think that it treats a chronic migraine-specific comorbidity that is invariably present in this condition—namely, the associated tightness of the neck, shoulder, and upper back muscles.

Several studies have shown that it is not beneficial in episodic migraine, and I think that this is the underlying reason. My impression is that in chronic migraine, the muscle tightness drives the frequency of the headaches and, consequently, accounts for its high headache frequency. Botulinum toxin is a very effective and long-lasting muscle relaxant, and I started employing it as such in the early nineties, when I was still performing trigger point injections.

The only botulinum toxin regimen with shown benefit in the treatment of chronic migraine involves thirty-one injections of five units each. We administer seven in the forehead, four in each temple, six in the back of the head, four in the back of the neck, and three in each shoulder. We conduct the injections with tiny needles, and although the procedure is not pleasant, it should not be painful either.

With botulinum toxin treatment of chronic migraine, it easily takes ten to fourteen days before we see the benefit; unfortunately, it often already wears off two to three weeks before the next set of injections is due, which is quarterly. In my experience, the overall benefit in chronic migraine is generally not as impressive as that of the CGRP antibodies.

The most common side effect I have encountered with botulinum toxin treatment of chronic migraine is soreness or weakness of the muscles in the back of the neck. If the patient reports neck weakness in particular, I am inclined to skip the back of the neck when I perform the injections.

Instead, I may use the remaining botulinum toxin to relax the jaw muscles, which are often tight as well in chronic migraine patients. My impression is that relaxing those muscles can contribute substantially to its migraine preventive benefit. I may inject them with fifteen or twenty botulinum toxin units each, palpating for taut bands in the muscles that I inject.

Chapter 12

What Do I Do When Pregnant?

Birth Control

Since the middle of the last century, medicine has made tremendous progress in developing ways to regulate pregnancy through hormonal birth control, a great invention that allows reliable family planning by very successfully preventing conception. For a long time, estrogen-containing birth control was the standard, but this has gradually changed and moved to progestin-only birth control, with tremendous additional benefits to women's health, including headaches.

However, before this change occurred, the estrogen dose in birth control progressively decreased from as high as 150 micrograms of mestranol, which is the equivalent of approximately 100 micrograms of estradiol, to as low as 10 micrograms of estradiol. What made this possible was the growing understanding that the contraceptive benefit of estrogen-containing birth control did not derive from the estrogen component but, instead, from its progestin content.

While estrogens suppress ovulation, progestins change the mucus in the entrance to the uterus, the cervix, in such a way that sperm cannot penetrate it. Consequently, suppression of ovulation is not necessary for effective birth control, as was initially thought.

Along with the design of the birth control as three weeks on and one week off, the estrogen component causes a bleeding in the week off, mimicking menstruation. Traditionally, women had been looking at menstruation as a beacon of reassurance that no pregnancy had occurred in the interim; hence, those who developed the birth control considered a monthly vaginal bleeding important from a psychological perspective. However, this has changed over time as well with the increasing confidence in the efficacy of hormonal birth control and the ubiquitous availability of pregnancy tests.

The lowering of the estrogen dose and, ultimately, the removal of the hormone altogether has been of significant benefit to women's health, in particular related to blood clotting disorders, such as deep vein thrombosis and lung embolism. The latter is a condition in which blood clots travel from the legs or pelvis to the lungs and cause symptoms, such as shortness of breath, chest pain, and cough.

In addition, estrogens increase the woman's risk of heart attack, stroke or brain attack, and breast cancer, even in the relatively low dosages as employed for menopausal estrogen therapy. Particularly relevant here is the negative effect of estrogens on headaches, both in terms of their frequency and intensity. Accordingly, I have seen the discontinuation of menopausal estrogen therapy impacting headaches in such a way that my services as a headache physician were no longer required.

Women who experience headaches, or the worsening thereof, on estrogen-containing birth control are generally not that lucky when they discontinue it. Certainly, their headaches may improve but, in my experience, never to the extent that they no longer need my services even if headaches were not their problem prior.

The strongest indication that the new-onset or worse headaches are due to the birth control is when they happen during the week off, along with the occurrence of the vaginal bleeding. I have seen physicians and other health care practitioners argue that these headaches cannot be from the birth control, because they happen during the week off.

This is faulty reasoning because they occur as a result of estrogen withdrawal, typically simultaneously with the vaginal bleeding. Estrogen withdrawal is probably one of the most potent headache triggers, if not the most potent one, and not only of headaches in general but also of migraine headaches.

Pregnancy

Although the estrogen level in the blood steadily increases during pregnancy to peak in the third trimester, headaches ordinarily improve; as far as I am concerned, this should be the expectation as part of the physiological changes of pregnancy. It means that when preexisting headaches, including migraine, do not improve or, worse, if they deteriorate or if there is new onset headache or the onset of a new type of headache, we should assume that something is amiss.

The general concern is that something is wrong neurologically, which means something bad is happening to the brain, and physicians or other health care practitioners end up referring the pregnant woman to a neurologist. I think that this is unfortunate, because neurologists only consider the possibility of brain disease causing or worsening the headaches of pregnancy, ignoring the potential medical causes.

This does not mean that the neurological causes are not important, which they are, but they are rare, and I believe that their significance stands in no proportion to the medical causes. Unfortunately, very little information is available about the non-neurological causes of pregnancy-related headaches, whether it is a lack of improvement or worsening of preexisting headaches, new onset headache, or the onset of a new type of headache.

This paucity of information reflects an absence of study derived from a lack of interest, which is the more amazing if you consider that worldwide, there are over 200 million pregnancies each year, of which, by the way, an estimated half are unintended.

Many things change during pregnancy, extending well beyond the exterior of the body; in fact, the internal changes related to the body's physiology are the most pronounced. In this regard, I already mentioned the rising blood estrogen level that peaks in the third trimester, which you would expect to worsen headache, given the negative impact of estrogens on headaches in general. Why this does not happen—in fact, as I strongly believe, we should expect headaches to improve during a normally developing pregnancy—we do not know.

A number of other changes that occur simultaneously may be relevant here. The first one is the cessation of ovulation and, hence, the elimination of the menstrual estrogen cycle. As mentioned, estrogens are bad for headaches; as it appears from clinical practice, especially when they fluctuate and more so when, with the fluctuation, they go down.

Another relevant hormonal change may be the steady increase in blood progesterone level that very much parallels that of the estrogen level. Both hormones are important for the normal functioning of the female body, pregnant or not, and work together.

However, some believe that progesterone mitigates the potentially negative effects of estrogens on the body, such as related to premenstrual syndrome, or PMS, which includes headaches. How this exactly works, nobody knows; when I researched it myself, treating patients with migraine headaches related to their menstrual cycle with progesterone, the results were disappointing.

A third change is the increase in thyroid function that happens during pregnancy, which I think is the most important one in the context of the well-being of the pregnant woman. In addition to the thyroid-stimulating hormone, or TSH, stimulating the thyroid gland to release its hormones, a hormone from the placenta, called human chorionic gonadotropin, or HCG, does very much the same.

The placenta forms within one to two weeks of conception, and almost as soon as it is established, it starts to release this hormone, also referred to as the pregnancy hormone. At the end of the first trimester, the placenta gains yet another important function, which is to provide oxygen and nutrients to the growing baby and remove waste products from its blood, allowing the baby to grow and prosper.

General Health

I think that it is nature's intention to put the pregnant woman in an excellent state of physical and mental health for the benefit of the developing baby, and that it does so mainly through the human chorionic gonadotropin hormone, or HCG, stimulating the thyroid gland. This should make her feel better, if not much better, in the course of the first trimester, and headache relief, I opine, is part of this improvement.

If it does not happen and the woman does not feel better coming out of the first trimester and, certainly, if she feels worse than before the pregnancy, several things should be considered, and thyroid function is high on the list.

During pregnancy, we determine thyroid function by measuring the level of thyroid-stimulating hormone, or TSH, in the blood; measuring the free levothyroxine, or FT4, level is not reliable because of other thyroid-related changes. It is important that we interpret the result against a trimester-specific reference range, preferably one for the local population representative of the patient.

This reference range should solely originate from the testing of pregnant women; only of those who are free of thyroid disease, have optimal iodine intake, and test negative for thyroid peroxidase antibody, or TPO-a. In the absence of such a specific reference range, a generally accepted upper limit of the blood thyroid-stimulating hormone level is 2.5 micro-international units per liter in the first trimester and 3.0 micro-international units per liter in the second and third trimesters.

Specifically in pregnancy, it is important to determine the level of thyroid peroxidase antibody as well when the blood thyroid-stimulating hormone level is borderline elevated. If the antibody level is positive, it is an additional reason to initiate treatment with levothyroxine, which is the standard treatment of low thyroid function, or hypothyroidism.

In order to secure good iodine availability to support the increase in thyroid function that is so vital to pregnancy, the American Thyroid Association recommends the daily intake of 150 micrograms of iodine as potassium iodide, commencing three months in advance of the pregnancy. Of course, the latter is only possible if the pregnancy is planned!

Low thyroid function, or hypothyroidism, is one of the four most common medical conditions that prevents a woman's health from improving and from being excellent during pregnancy. The other three are low hemoglobin, or anemia, characterized by a shortage of red blood cells, diabetes mellitus, and high blood pressure, or hypertension.

Of those four, all except diabetes potentially negatively impact headaches, either preventing them from getting better, making them worse, or causing new onset headache or a new type of headache. They happen each in as many as one out of twenty pregnancies, are easy to detect, and can be treated effectively with little intervention and at low cost. Therefore, it is important to consider them from the onset of pregnancy to the end, especially if it does not progress as desired, no matter whether headaches are part of that or not.

Brain Disease

In rare instances, pregnancy-related headaches are due to a disorder affecting the brain, for which neurological consultation is appropriate. These conditions almost exclusively occur during the third trimester or in the six weeks following delivery, which we refer to as puerperium.

An exception is idiopathic intracranial hypertension, or IIH, also called pseudotumor cerebri or benign intracranial hypertension. Although its risk is not elevated during pregnancy, if it does develop, this is most likely to happen during the first or second trimester. Generalized headaches, generally of low-grade intensity, are the cardinal symptom, associated with visual complaints due to swelling of the optic discs.

The optic disc is the site in the back of the eye, or eye ground, where the optic nerve enters the eye. As it is an extension of the brain, the optic nerve and, consequently, the optic disc swells when the brain swells, which is the problem in idiopathic intracranial hypertension.

We do not know why the brain swells in this particular condition, but sometimes it is due to a blood clot in one of the big veins that drain blood from the brain. The likelihood of this is increased during pregnancy, as well as during the three months afterward, because of a fivefold elevated risk of developing blood clots.

The swelling of the optic discs is easy to detect with an examination of the eye grounds called fundoscopy. A special type of magnetic resonance imaging (MRI) of the brain, a so-called brain venogram, can reveal whether the brain swelling is due to a blood clot in a vein.

A brain disorder of pregnancy related to the development of high blood pressure, or hypertension, is eclampsia, which is characterized by the occurrence of seizures. Generalized headaches typically precede this condition by days or weeks, typically associated with pain in the right-upper abdomen due to enlargement of the liver and swelling of the feet and lower legs due to edema. It merely requires measuring the blood pressure and testing for protein in the urine to diagnose; treating the hypertension prevents the seizures.

A stroke, or brain attack, can occur during pregnancy as well, but that is very rare. From a headache perspective, undoubtedly most dramatic is what we refer to as a subarachnoid hemorrhage. This is a bleeding between the two inner membranes surrounding the brain, caused by the rupture of an aneurysm, which is a localized expansion of an artery that looks like a little balloon.

It causes a headache that comes on like a blow to the head—that is, a headache of very acute or peracute onset, also referred to as thunderclap headache. It is a medical emergency, because half of the people who suffer from such a bleed unfortunately die. The risk of a subarachnoid hemorrhage happening during pregnancy is not higher than otherwise, but it can occur nevertheless.

Two other types of strokes, or brain attacks, can also happen during pregnancy, caused by the blockage of an artery or a vein. An artery is a blood vessel that carries blood from the heart—in this case, to the brain and veins, in turn bring it back from the brain to the heart. In general, strokes are due to a blood clot obstructing a brain artery; during pregnancy, however, this is more likely to impact a vein because of the increased tendency of the blood to clot.

As a result, strokes in pregnancy or afterward, during puerperium, are more likely to present with headaches, which can be severe, and with seizures. When the stroke is from a blocked artery, headaches are less common and generally low-grade and, thus, not particularly intense. Under such circumstances, stroke most often affects the back of the brain, where vision is located, resulting in loss of vision on one side or the other.

Investigation

When it comes to headaches and pregnancy, as mentioned, the expectation should be that they get better, along with the improvement in the woman's general health, certainly toward the end of the first trimester. If this does not happen and they remain the same and, definitely, if they worsen, it should be assumed that something is amiss, and proper investigation should follow.

The most common reasons are medical, not neurological, and require such simple examinations as measuring the blood pressure and testing the blood for anemia and low thyroid function, or hypothyroidism. If necessary, these simple investigations should be repeated during the pregnancy, because a change over time is much more informative than a single measurement. For this reason, it is important as well to have baseline values, which of course is only possible if the pregnancy is planned.

If there is new onset headache or the onset of a new type of headache, the same should be done with a medical evaluation first and a neurological consultation second unless the headache is of peracute onset, like a blow to the head. Of course, the same is true if the headaches are associated with neurological symptoms, such as seizures, suggesting either eclampsia or a so-called venous stroke from obstruction of a vein.

It goes without saying that neurological complaints are always worrisome regardless of whether headaches are present or not and, if present, even when the headaches are mild. Those symptoms can be one-sided face drooping, one-sided arm weakness or numbness, one-sided loss of vision, or difficulty speaking. Otherwise, it is important to look for a medical cause first, which is easy to do and does not involve a lot of effort or cost.

Treatment

If the pregnant woman is healthy and the medical evaluation is unrevealing, her headaches should be treated as migraine unless there is a specific reason to do otherwise. As with migraine in general, the first step is to secure effective abortive treatment, defined as treatment that *fully* relieves the headaches within two hours and does so consistently and without side effects.

Obstetricians and midwives still have a tendency to prescribe barbiturate-containing or opioid medications, which are addicting and may negatively impact the development of the baby's brain. I strongly recommend the use of sumatriptan instead, a specific abortive migraine medication with which we have over three decades experience. The latter extends well beyond clinical practice and includes a large pregnancy registry and several well-conducted pregnancy studies.

The medication is available in four formulations—namely, oral tablet, nasal spray, subcutaneous injection, and rectal suppository, the latter only in Europe. The sumatriptan tablet comes in three strengths, 25, 50, and 100 milligrams; the regular liquid nasal spray in two strengths, 5 and 20 milligrams; the injection in three strengths, 3, 4, and 6 milligrams; and the suppository in two strengths, 12.5 and 25 milligrams.

The sumatriptan nasal spray is also marketed in a powder formulation and as a liquid nasal spray with a membrane permeability enhancer, both with better absorption and, possibly, better efficacy. Of all those formulations and dosages, however, I mostly prescribe the one-hundred-milligram tablet and the three-milligram or four-milligram subcutaneous injection.

If the woman can treat the headaches at mild or mild-to-moderate intensity, I prescribe half of the one-hundred-milligram tablet, repeated after two hours if the headache is not fully relieved. If she generally needs to repeat the medication to obtain full headache relief and tolerates it well, I will have her take the whole tablet. If she can treat at moderate or moderate-to-severe headache intensity only, I prescribe the one-hundred-milligram tablet, which she can repeat after two hours if it does not provide full headache relief.

If she cannot initiate treatment until the headache is severe, she will require the sumatriptan injection, if necessary repeated after an hour, or use a sumatriptan tablet to relieve residual headache, if present. Patients generally tolerate the medication well; potential side effects include tingling in the fingers, tightness in the upper chest or throat, and nausea.

In case the frequency of the headaches is such that it requires preventive treatment, we should consider medications the very last resort. If the neck, shoulder, and upper back muscles are tight, which is almost invariably the case, especially with frequently occurring headaches, she should use a heating pad twice daily on the muscles for fifteen to twenty minutes each time.

We can add gentle massage, or alternatively, she can combine the daily use of the heating pad with a relaxation exercise, also to promote rest. If the jaw muscles are tight, there is an indication for a mouth guard to relax the muscles, prevent clenching and grinding, called bruxism, and protect the structure of the teeth.

If fatigue is an issue, assuring uninterrupted sleep at night of sufficient duration and encouraging napping during the day are important measures to take—of course, after ascertaining that anemia, iron deficiency, or hypothyroidism are not the cause of the fatigue. We may be able to improve sleep with nonprescription medications, such as valerian, melatonin, or diphenhydramine. Nausea or reflux we can treat with calcium carbonate and constipation with docusate or magnesium citrate.

When it comes to medications for migraine prevention, during pregnancy we should use them only if absolutely necessary. We should avoid beta-blockers unless to treat hypertension and prevent eclampsia, because they increase the risk of preterm delivery and low birth weight. Of the tricyclics, we know through numerous studies that they do not increase the risk of miscarriage, preterm delivery, low birth weight, or congenital abnormalities.

For use during pregnancy, we prefer nortriptyline, should not prescribe imipramine, and should use amitriptyline only if sedation is required to improve sleep. Effective dosages of the tricyclics usually lie between twenty-five and seventy-five milligrams with the medication taken once daily at bedtime or two hours before, if falling asleep is a problem. The most common side effects are dry mouth, constipation, increased appetite, and weight gain.

Chapter 13

What Is Cluster Headache?

Presentation

Cluster headache is a headache disorder related to migraine in the sense that it runs in the same families. It is rare, however, certainly in comparison to migraine, which affects as much as 15 percent of the population; it is about one hundred times less common.

In contrast to migraine, which affects women two to three times more often than men, cluster headache is almost entirely limited to men. Also, as opposed to migraine, it almost exclusively concerns adults, although I have seen it in a boy as young as six years old.

The headaches in cluster headache are usually severe or very severe in intensity and last much less time than migraine headaches do but are definitely as incapacitating. They come on quickly, building to their maximum intensity in five to ten minutes, last one to two hours, and disappear as quickly as they appear. They occur daily or almost daily, often two or three times per twenty-four hours, with a predilection for the night.

At night, they wake the patient from sleep; generally, this happens between midnight and two o'clock in the morning. In migraine, this is different; if headaches do occur nocturnally, they usually wake the patient from sleep between four and six o'clock in the morning.

Nocturnal Migraine

Headaches that wake the patient from sleep at night are relatively rare in migraine and only do so when severe. It becomes more common as we get older, and in some older migraineurs, the headaches predominantly happen this way—that is, nocturnally. When this is the case, they often occur relatively frequently, easily several times per week, and we need to differentiate it from chronic migraine.

We need to distinguish it from chronic migraine even when, due to the high frequency, the total headache burden is half a month or more, because the treatment is different. I refer to this particular migraine presentation as nocturnal migraine, and the treatment is similar to that of cluster headache, which makes it appropriate to discuss that here. The following patient vignette is an example of nocturnal migraine.

A sixty-nine-year-old woman has been experiencing headaches since the age of fourteen, when she started menstruating. Since their onset, they have been severe. When she was in her mid-twenties, the headaches occurred three or four times per week; for the last twenty-five to thirty years, they have been almost daily.

The headaches wake her from sleep between two and four o'clock in the morning 85 percent of the time, being 8/10 in intensity. In the remaining 15 percent, they come on during the day, but not at any particular time. The diurnal headaches are 7–8/10 in intensity and build to their maximum intensity in a half hour to an hour.

The headaches last six to eight hours but can continue for as long as a day. They are located in the left temple or across the forehead. The headaches are sharp, steady in nature, and when severe, they are associated with photophobia and phonophobia. In approximately a quarter, the headaches are associated with nausea as well.

Location

The pain in cluster headache is always limited to the right or left side of the head and is typically located in or behind the eye. It rarely switches sides, which means that it is generally side-locked. This is different from migraine, where the pain is limited to the right or left side in approximately two-thirds of patients and typically does switch sides. I look for the latter in the history of the patient, because it reassures me that the headaches are not caused by a brain abnormality.

If due to a brain disorder, the patient experiences the headaches on the side of the abnormality or on both sides; if one-sided or unilateral, they do not switch sides. When headaches switch sides, as in migraine, it is important that the side they switch from is pain-free. If this is not the case, the headaches are not unilateral; they involve the other side of the head as well and, hence, are bilateral.

The location of one-sided migraine headaches is typically in the temple, extending into the eye when the pain increases in intensity. In general, the more forward the pain reaches, the more intense the headache. Pain in the temple is typically of a pulsating, throbbing, or pounding nature. In contrast, pain in the eye is generally sharp like a dagger; it can also be like an intense pressure, which feels as if pushing the eye out of the socket.

When the eye becomes involved in headache, it often acts up in other ways as well, such as turning red, which we call conjunctival injection, and starting to tear, referred to as lacrimation. This happens particularly in cluster headache, probably because of the high intensity of the pain. The upper eyelid may droop, called ptosis, the pupil can narrow, known as miosis, and the area around the eye may become puffy, or edematous. The nose can also get involved, and the nostril on the side of the pain may become congested and can run as well, called rhinorrhea.

It is important to remember that those complaints, which we refer to as autonomic symptoms, are neither specific to cluster headache nor necessary for the diagnosis, as people often assume.

Diagnosis

We diagnose cluster headache exclusively on the pattern of occurrence of the headaches, which means headaches that happen daily or almost daily, several times per day, particularly at night, and lasting one to two hours. In between, there is no pain, although occasionally, there may be a mild, lingering background pain.

As mentioned, the headaches are always on the right or left side of the head only—that is, unilateral—and stay there, not switching sides. They are typically located in or behind the eye but can extend upward into the forehead or downward into the cheek.

Eye and nose symptoms, as outlined above, can be present, but they do not have to be, and their appearance does not diagnose the condition. Once again, it is the temporal pattern, as we call it, of the headaches that dictates the diagnosis, nothing more and nothing less.

When they occur at night, the headaches typically wake the patient from sleep in the early hours of the night, usually between midnight and two o'clock. With migraine headaches, if this happens, it is usually in the early morning hours—that is, between four and six o'clock.

While migraineurs want to remain motionless with their headaches and, if possible, recline with the head slightly elevated, cluster headache patients cannot keep still and feel compelled to move. Consequently, if the headaches occur at night, which is usually the case, they get up from bed and pace the floor restlessly. They may also behave somewhat violently, such as rocking the body or banging the head against the wall.

Restless behavior like that is unlikely in migraineurs, although on one occasion, I saw a migraine patient in the hospital come out of bed when the headache became excruciatingly severe and pace the floor. I think that this difference in behavior is because, in contrast to migraineurs, cluster headache patients generally are not nauseated with their headaches.

It is often the development of nausea as the headache progresses in intensity that disables the migraine patient. Although the headache is sensitive to movement as well, any kind of motion aggravates the nausea and may even evoke an acute spell of vomiting.

The headaches in cluster headache generally occur daily or almost daily and several times per day for weeks or months, to be gone for months or sometimes even years. This clustering of the headaches is what gave it its current name, which we had previously known under a variety of terms, such as histaminic cephalalgia, migrainous neuralgia, and Horton's headache. On a historical note, it was a neurologist from Portland, Maine, by the name of E. Charles Kunkle, who coined the term *cluster headache* in 1952.

Currently, we call the condition episodic cluster headache if the headaches happen in the clustering pattern described above; we refer to it as chronic cluster headache if such clusters do not or do no longer occur. The clusters themselves we call episodes, and the headache-free periods between them we refer to as remissions.

Clusters should not be confused with flurries, which we sometimes see in migraine with aura. In those, several attacks happen during a one- or two-week period, and then there are no attacks for months. The below patient vignettes are examples of the episodic and chronic presentations of cluster headache.

A twenty-nine-year-old man has been experiencing headaches since the age of twenty-four, which is shortly after he got married. They last an hour and occur once or twice per day, usually in the early morning or late evening, building to their maximum intensity in five minutes. The headaches are located on the right—in the eye, temple, and back of the head and neck.

They are associated with light sensitivity and blurred vision of the right eye. The eye also tears, the right nostril runs, and his stomach feels queasy. The headaches happen in episodes, lasting four to six weeks with remissions of up to a year.

A thirty-four-year-old man has been experiencing headaches since the age of twenty-three. They last twenty minutes to two hours and occur daily, once or twice per day. The headaches usually come on in the early night, waking him from sleep. They are located on the left—in the temple and the cheek.

The headaches are associated with tearing of the left eye and congestion of the left nostril. Alcohol and daytime napping bring them on. In addition, the headaches appear more often during hot and humid weather. They are worse lying down and make him pace the floor. The headaches happen in episodes, lasting two to four weeks with remissions of twelve to fifteen months.

A twenty-nine-year-old man has been experiencing headaches since the age of nine or ten. Initially, they occurred once every few months; for the last five years, the headaches have been daily. They last a half hour to two hours and happen one to six times per day with an average of two. The headaches only occasionally wake him from sleep at night.

They are located in the right eye, forehead, temple, and cheek, with the maximum pain felt behind the eye. The eye turns red, tears, and is very sensitive to light while the right nostril becomes congested. During the headaches, he is usually able to function, but he lies down if he can. Alcohol brings them on in thirty minutes.

A forty-three-year-old man has been experiencing headaches since the age of thirty-eight. They occurred daily for three months, followed by a remission of eight months, and then again daily for five months, followed by a remission of eight months. For the last three years, the headaches have been daily without remission. They last one to two hours and happen four or five times per day.

The headaches come on any time during the day and wake him from sleep at night as well. They build to their maximum intensity in fifteen minutes. The headaches are located behind the left eye and in the left-hand back of the neck. They are very severe in intensity and throbbing in nature. Reddening, tearing, and light sensitivity of the left eye accompany the headaches, as well as perspiration of the scalp.

Treatment

Regarding the treatment of cluster headache, the lifestyle recommendations are limited to two: no napping during the day and no alcohol. However, both are relevant only when the headaches are active, which for the patient with episodic cluster headache means during the episodes. Then, even a small amount of alcohol brings on a headache, typically in thirty to forty-five minutes. This happens so consistently that I have noticed that patients sometimes use it to see whether they are in remission. Generally, however, they know when they are.

Other than these two lifestyle recommendations, the treatment of cluster headache is with medications, or pharmacological. In contrast to migraine, we initiate abortive and preventive treatment at the same time. In migraine, we start with abortive treatment, consider the general health of the patient, and add preventive treatment if indicated. With cluster headache, both treatments are necessary and initiated simultaneously because of the high intensity and high frequency of the headaches.

For the abortive treatment of cluster headache, the sumatriptan injection is by far the most effective; it is even more efficacious here than in migraine. In cluster headache, it fully relieves a headache that is even very severe in five to ten minutes while in migraine, this generally takes twenty to forty minutes.

As in migraine, I usually start with the three-milligram or four-milligram dose, because the patient can administer it up to three or four times per day, keeping in mind that the maximum daily dose is twelve milligrams. However, if the benefit is not as desired, I increase the dose to six milligrams, which the patient can use up to twice per twenty-four hours.

Particularly with the six-milligram dose, we can expect side effects, although cluster headache patients generally tolerate medications much better than migraine patients do. Most common is a rush that ascends in the body to the upper chest, neck, and face, very much like a hot flash—usually lasting no longer than five to ten minutes, however. It can be associated with a sensation of pressure or tightness in the upper chest, throat, back of the neck, or head, which can also appear instead.

Sumatriptan is a potent vasoconstrictor, especially when administered by injection, and we should not prescribe it to patients with uncontrolled or poorly controlled hypertension, cardiovascular disease, or cerebrovascular disease.

An alternative is the inhalation of 100 percent oxygen, but nowadays, it is rare that I still prescribe this. It requires an oxygen tank and a special so-called non-rebreather mask that allows for the delivery of highly concentrated oxygen. It is a particular mask with circles of little holes on each side, and it is important that valves are present to cover those holes. Otherwise, too much air enters the mask on breathing in, diluting the oxygen and making it much less effective.

The patient should use the oxygen with the non-rebreather mask for ten to twenty minutes at the onset of headache at a rate of eight to ten liters per minute. It can be ideal for nocturnal attacks with the tank stored in the bedroom where people generally do not smoke. Smoking is a notorious explosion hazard in the presence of oxygen!

Treatment with oxygen remains quite a hassle, however, certainly in comparison to the sumatriptan injection. The latter is obviously much easier to administer, and the benefit is generally faster in onset and more profound.

Preventive Treatment

The treatment of choice for preventing cluster headache attacks used to be verapamil, and I developed the high-dose therapy specifically for this purpose. Importantly, we execute this particular treatment with long-acting tablets, also referred to as extended-release or sustained-release tablets, taken twice daily and approximately twelve hours apart.

I start with 120 milligrams, sustained release, twice daily and increase the dose after a week to 240 milligrams, sustained release, twice daily. In episodic cluster headache, this may be sufficient to prevent the headaches. If not, I order an electrocardiogram, or ECG, and look at the electrical conduction in the heart, called atrioventricular, or AV, conduction. If it is fine, I increase the dose to 240 milligrams in the morning and 360 milligrams in the evening. I prefer to prescribe the highest dose in the evening because of the tendency of cluster headache attacks to happen at night.

The goal of preventive cluster headache treatment is to abolish the headaches fully, which means that I will further increase the dose if required. This is usually not needed in episodic cluster headache, but in chronic cluster headache, it is generally necessary to further uptitrate the dose.

In such cases, I increase the verapamil by 120 milligrams, sustained release, per day with weekly intervals, followed by another electrocardiogram after each dose increase to monitor the atrioventricular conduction. In patients with chronic cluster headache, I have gone up as high as 960 or 1,200 milligrams per day, again and very importantly, using sustained-release tablets only.

It is paramount to discontinue the verapamil once the patient is out of an episode, because it does not prevent another one from occurring. If we continue it and another episode happens, we will have to further increase the dose. We will have to do that in order to get the headaches under control, and there is a limit as to how high we can uptitrate it.

The most common side effect of verapamil is constipation, commonly seen with its use for migraine prevention. However, I do not believe that I have ever encountered it in patients with cluster headache, even with the very high dosages I sometimes employ.

What I have seen occasionally is swelling of the feet when the patient ends up on a very high dose. A small amount of a water tablet, or diuretic, like 25 milligrams of hydrochlorothiazide, or HCTZ, generally solves the problem. We should not use verapamil when heart disease is present or when there is an issue with the electrical conduction in the heart.

If we have a patient with chronic cluster headache and we cannot prevent the headaches fully with verapamil, adding a small dose of lithium—for example, three hundred milligrams per day—can be helpful. We can also employ the lithium alone in those patients, but I have not done that for a long time, preferring to combine it with verapamil.

If we need to bring the headaches rapidly under control because they are very intense or very frequent, we can do so with a course of a corticosteroid, like prednisone. I always give it in four divided dosages, taken with meals and at bedtime with a snack to protect the stomach. I start with sixty milligrams per day for three days, after which I decrease it by five milligrams per day every two days, starting with the morning dose.

This slow prednisone taper provides a twenty-five-day schedule and requires 170 tablets in total, five milligrams each. As soon as I start it, I also always initiate preventive treatment that we can, if needed, maintain for a longer period. Depending on the patient, I may add stomach protection as well, usually in the form of a proton-pump inhibitor, or PPI, like omeprazole, twenty milligrams, or lansoprazole, fifteen milligrams, once or twice daily.

CGRP Antibody

One of the CGRP antibodies, galcanezumab, we studied not only for migraine prevention but also in cluster headache and found it effective in the episodic presentation of the condition. However, we prescribed it in a different dose—namely, not 120 milligrams but 300 milligrams subcutaneously monthly.

For this purpose, it is available in prefilled syringes, each containing one hundred milligrams. We administer three of those injections under the skin, or subcutaneously, preferably in the abdomen, and do so monthly as long as the headaches occur. This has become my preventive treatment of choice in episodic cluster headache because of its benign nature and ease of use.

Like for migraine prevention, galcanezumab does not have listed side effects in cluster headache other than injection site reactions. In addition, it does not interact with other medications, which means that there are no biologic-drug or biologic-biologic interactions. It does not have contraindications, meaning circumstances under which we cannot prescribe it. It also does not require building up the dose, that is uptitration, and we do not have to adjust the dose in case of liver or kidney disease.

It is unfortunate that the study of galcanezumab in chronic cluster headache patients did not show benefit. In my opinion, however, this does not mean that it does not work preventively in those patients. My concern is that the study included many patients with what we call symptomatic cluster headache.

These are patients with headaches resembling cluster headache but of a different origin. I have seen numerous of them in practice, and the cause resides commonly in the nose-sinus system. Originating there, the eye and nose symptoms are present that we associate with cluster headache, leading to the erroneous diagnosis.

The key distinguishing feature is that those patients are not free of pain between the attacks that resemble cluster headache. The persistent pain is generally not in the eye, where the headaches are located, but in the side of the nose or in the cheek. Intranasal contact is often the cause, with the exacerbations that resemble cluster headache attacks felt in or behind the eye.

Symptomatic cluster headache is much less common, if existent at all, in episodic cluster headache because of its episodic nature. This particular pattern of headache occurrence is not compatible with a structural cause, in the same way as alternating headaches that are sometimes on the left and sometimes on the right, are not compatible with brain disease.

Chapter 14

What Are Rare Headache Conditions?

Stabbing Headache

Cluster headache is a headache disorder that affects approximately one person in a thousand. This makes it quite rare, but there are even less common headache conditions that are worth mentioning here. However, before delving into them, I would like to elaborate on a type of headache that is not well-known although it is not that rare and can be scary to experience.

We refer to it as stabbing headache, ice pick headache, or jabs and jolts, a sharp, jabbing pain that strikes the head like lightning, lasting seconds but sometimes with an after-pain lingering for one to two minutes. It is intense to the extent that it makes you grab your head or hold your breath.

Such headaches are relatively common in patients with migraine or cluster headache, but they generally have them only occasionally. People not otherwise affected by headaches sometimes also experience them and may have them regularly or even frequently. In practice, I have seen patients with these headaches suffer from them daily, several hundred times per day.

Even when they occur occasionally, they often make people worry that something ominous is going on in their head, like a brain artery ballooning into an aneurysm that may burst. However, nothing of that kind is happening, because no brain abnormality manifests itself in this particular way.

We used to treat stabbing headache with indomethacin, which is a powerful nonsteroidal anti-inflammatory drug, or NSAID. It is also very potent in upsetting the stomach; hence, we either do not prescribe it anymore or combine it with a proton-pump inhibitor, or PPI, to protect the stomach.

If I prescribe it, I generally do so in a sustained-release formulation that contains seventy-five milligrams of the medication. I give one of those capsules in the morning at breakfast and a regular twenty-five-milligram capsule in the evening at bedtime or, instead, prescribe the seventy-five-milligram sustained-release capsule twice daily at breakfast and at dinner. In order to protect the stomach, I combine each seventy-five-milligram capsule with a medication like omeprazole in a dose of twenty milligrams taken along with it.

As we often encounter stabbing headache in patients with migraine or cluster headache, we think that the underlying mechanism is similar. Consequently, we can also treat it with a regular preventive migraine medication, such as a beta-blocker or one that targets the CGRP pathway, like a gepant or CGRP antibody.

Indomethacin

Indomethacin is an interesting medication because it is not only a potent nonsteroidal anti-inflammatory pain medication, or analgesic. As a vasoconstrictor, it narrows the blood vessels in the head, although mildly, and as a vasodilator, it slightly widens the blood vessels in the rest of the body.

We studied it in the 1970s as an abortive migraine medication in the form of a rectal suppository, because when taken by mouth, its absorption from the small bowel into the blood is quite slow. For a medication like that to be effective, it has to get absorbed into the blood fast—the faster, the better.

The rectum provides a good surface for the rapid absorption of medications and better than, for example, the lining of the nose. However, it is not terribly convenient in usage, to say the least. The indomethacin suppository proved effective, and before the advent of the triptans, I prescribed it regularly to my patients. It is a relatively effective headache or migraine medication, because it combines potent pain relief, or analgesia, with anti-inflammation and mild vasoconstriction.

Prior to the triptans, I used one thousand milligrams of water-soluble aspirin as the first line of treatment, after pretreatment with ten milligrams of metoclopramide to promote the absorption of the aspirin and to prevent nausea. As the second line, I prescribed the indomethacin rectal suppository either in a dose of fifty milligrams, repeated every half hour, or in a dose of one hundred milligrams, repeated every hour, until full headache relief and with a maximum of two hundred milligrams per day.

As the third line of treatment, I used the ergotamine-caffeine suppository that contained two milligrams of ergotamine and one hundred milligrams of caffeine. I prescribed it in a dose of one-third suppository every hour until the headache was fully relieved and with a maximum of two suppositories per day.

I did not employ these three lines of treatment sequentially, however, as in step care, in which the potency of treatment is gradually increased and of which I am not a proponent. I used them in a targeted way depending on the intensity of the headaches at the time of treatment, their speed of development, and their duration.

The most common side effect of the indomethacin suppository was light-headedness when getting up too quickly from lying down due to its vasodilatory effect in the body. The most common side effect of the ergotamine-caffeine suppository was nausea, and because of it, the patient administered only one-third of a suppository at a time and repeated it, if necessary, with intervals of an hour.

Absolute Response

We have two headache conditions—paroxysmal hemicrania and hemicrania continua—that uniquely respond to preventive treatment with indomethacin. Both have a so-called absolute response to it. This means that the headaches are fully, 100 percent, relieved when the medication is taken daily in an appropriate dose, which is usually between 100 and 150 milligrams per day. The benefit occurs overnight and persists for as long as the treatment is continued.

The two disorders are very rare, however, although some people claim differently. I have seen fewer than half a dozen of each in the course of more than four decades of dedicated headache practice. A neurologist from Norway, Professor Ottar Sjaastad, described paroxysmal hemicrania in 1974 as an indomethacin-responsive headache syndrome. Together with him, I described hemicrania continua as a similar syndrome in 1984, when I was a neurology resident in the Netherlands.

Paroxysmal Hemicrania

I consider paroxysmal hemicrania a variant of cluster headache, because its presentation is very similar. The difference is that in paroxysmal hemicrania, the headaches are even shorter in duration and happen even more frequently; they last ten to thirty minutes, as opposed to one to two hours in cluster headache, and occur at least half a dozen times, if not more, per twenty-four hours.

Also, in contrast to cluster headache, which is predominantly a male condition, paroxysmal hemicrania is, like migraine, more common in women. The following are patient vignettes of episodic and chronic paroxysmal hemicrania respectively.

A fifty-three-year-old man has been experiencing headaches since the age of thirty-eight. They happen in episodes that last five to ten days. Initially, the episodes occurred twice per year; over time, they increased in frequency to monthly. In each episode, the headaches start off as twinges of mild pain, which last a few minutes only.

The twinges happen as infrequently as once per day but rapidly increase in frequency, intensity, and duration. Within two or three days, the headaches are full-blown, last five to ten minutes, and occur every two hours with clocklike regularity, day and night. They are severe, build to their maximum intensity in less than a minute, and disappear as quickly as they come on.

The headaches are located in the left forehead and are sharp, steady in nature. The left eye is very sensitive to light and becomes red and teary; the lower eyelid swells slightly. The left nostril runs during the headaches but is not congested. The headaches are so intense that they make it impossible for him to work, and at night, they wake him from sleep.

During the headaches, he sits up in a chair as quietly as possible, preferably in a dark and quiet room. Lying down makes them worse because of sensitivity of the left-hand back of his head and neck. The headaches continue full-blown, as described, for four or five days. Then they rapidly decrease in frequency, intensity, and duration to disappear in two or three days. Indomethacin, twenty-five milligrams four times per day, fully abolished them.

A sixty-two-year-old woman has been experiencing headaches since adolescence. Until several years ago, they happened infrequently and only several times per year. Then the headaches rapidly increased in frequency and, over the course of a month, became daily. They occur two or three times during the day and three times at night, lasting twenty to thirty minutes.

The headaches are located in the right temple as a localized sharp, steady pain. When severe, they are associated with pressure behind the right eye. The headaches are also associated with slight redness and tearing of the right eye and running but no congestion of the right nostril.

During the headaches, a blood vessel swells up in the right temple, which expands further on bending over. Stiffness of the muscles in the right back of the neck precedes them by fifteen to twenty minutes. Alcohol brings on the headaches in ten to fifteen minutes, and they happen as well when she oversleeps.

Aspirin taken as needed in a dose of 650 or 1,000 milligrams is effective in relieving the headaches. On indomethacin, 75 milligrams sustained-release twice daily, they decreased in frequency from five or six to two times per twenty-four hours. Increasing the dose to 75 milligrams three times per day fully abolished them.

Hemicrania Continua

Hemicrania continua, although indomethacin responsive as well, is a very different headache condition from paroxysmal hemicrania. The only additional feature that the two share is that the headaches are limited to the right or left side of the head and do not shift sides, making them what we call unilateral and side-locked.

Hemicrania continua is a continuous, as opposed to paroxysmal, headache disorder with the headaches present daily and continuously without breaks, unless the patient takes aspirin or an aspirin-like medication. As is the case with paroxysmal hemicrania, aspirin has a wonderful effect on this headache condition despite the relatively high level intensity of the pain.

The aspirin responsiveness was what led me to prescribe indomethacin to the patient, who became one of the two that Professor Sjaastad and I described under the term *hemicrania continua*. I just looked at indomethacin as a super aspirin; it certainly had a super effect on the patient, fully relieving his headaches. The following patient vignette is another example of this very rare headache disorder.

A forty-eight-year-old woman has been experiencing headaches since her late teens. Initially, they happened twice per month, relieved by nonprescription pain medications. Over time, the headaches gradually increased in frequency and have been daily for the last two or three years. They are present on awakening in the morning, do not change in any particular way over the day, and do not wake her from sleep at night.

The headaches are located on the right—in the eye, forehead, side of the head, and back of the neck. They are steady, vicelike in nature and mostly moderate in intensity. The headaches are not associated with light or noise sensitivity, nausea, or vomiting. Bending over makes them worse, and lying down makes them somewhat better. The headaches are also worse with menstruation.

Her neck and shoulder muscles are tight and sore on the right, and her right arm is somewhat sore as well. She takes 1,000 to 1,500 milligrams of aspirin per day with 40 percent relief of the headaches. On indomethacin, 25 milligrams four times per day, she became virtually headache-free.

Unlike paroxysmal hemicrania, we cannot diagnose hemicrania continua based on its presentation, because it is rather nonspecific, as should also be evident from the above patient vignette. Many people have this kind of continuous headache limited to the right or left side of the head and do not benefit much, if at all, from aspirin or aspirin-like medications. Consequently, they will not respond to indomethacin with full resolution of their headaches, as required for the diagnosis. In addition, it should be clear that indomethacin-resistant hemicrania continua is not only an oxymoron but does not exist.

Finally, eye or nose symptoms, like redness, tearing, swelling, congestion, and running, are not necessary for the diagnosis. Similarly, they are not required for that of cluster headache or paroxysmal hemicrania, and they do not constitute a basis for those diagnoses either. Diagnostically, migraine does not become cluster headache, because the eye turns red and tears or because the nose becomes congested and runs. We diagnose these headache conditions based on the temporal pattern in which the headaches happen—that is, how they occur over time.

Chapter 15

Do I Have Headaches from a Concussion?

Neck Injury

Concussion is certainly a cause of headaches, which can be severe or even very severe, but in my opinion, it is not a likely instigator of chronic headaches. Head and neck injuries alike can cause concussion, the latter by forcefully moving the brain within the skull. While the head directly connects to the neck and vice versa, head and neck injuries do not necessarily always go together, although they often do.

If they do, the head generates much more pain than the neck, pushing the neck injury to the background. As a result, neck injuries associated with head injuries generally do not get the kind of attention they deserve, and I think that this is a problem when it comes to the development of chronic headaches.

Neck injuries that are not associated with head injuries may not give rise to headaches until days or weeks later with the often-ignored neck symptoms, such as tightness, stiffness, soreness, or pain, bridging the time gap.

The direction in which the injury occurs largely determines the extent to which the neck is injured. A frontal injury, whether getting hit from the front or falling to the front, generally brings about the worst injury to the head and the lightest to the neck. Such injuries have the highest rate and severity of concussions and the lowest rate of chronic headaches, due to the absence of stretching of the muscles in the back of the neck, called the posterior neck muscles or posterior cervical muscles.

Particularly rear and sidewise injuries cause stretching of the muscles in the back of the neck and, consequently, are much more likely to result in chronic headaches, whether the injury is from a hit or from a fall. Forceful bending, or flexion, of the neck can cause the stretching or, alternatively, it can cause a so-called whiplash injury.

The latter is the kind of injury—in this case, of the neck—in which the neck forcefully bends in one direction and then snaps back to the opposite side. If the whiplash injury happens from the back, often due to a rear-end car accident, the head is thrown back; it then snaps forward, which forcefully stretches the muscles in the back of the neck.

A similar type of movement occurs when the injury comes from the side. This often happens in car accidents as well, with the head first thrown to the side of the impact and then snapping back in the opposite direction. The ultimate injury to the neck muscles is on the side of the impact and is due to the forceful stretch caused by the head snapping back, away from the injury.

Muscles

Muscles do not tolerate forceful stretching well, which causes them to go into spasm, probably for reasons of self-protection. The unfortunate consequence is that they end up squeezing off their circulation, making it difficult for them to heal. That is why it is important to identify muscle injury as it occurs, recognize it as to its significance, and direct the treatment accordingly.

Generally, that is not what we do, however, and advise pain medications where we should be prescribing muscle relaxants and, in addition, whatever else is appropriate to remedy such an injury. In this regard, I recommend the daily use of a heating pad to relax the neck, shoulder, and upper back muscles and improve their circulation.

Relaxing the muscles and improving their circulation promotes healing from the stretch injury, which over time allows the muscles to resume normal function. If the neck muscles remain tight, this tightness eventually spreads to the head and causes headaches. It may pick up an existing vulnerability to migraine as well and, consequently, lead to intense headaches. It may also spread to involve the jaw muscles and generate face pain instead or in addition to the headaches.

Face pain is often associated with headaches, including migraine headaches, because tightness of jaw muscles generates headaches in the same way neck muscle tightness does. This is the reason I like to include the jaw muscles, if they are tight, when I treat a chronic migraine patient with botulinum toxin. I may do so instead of injecting the muscles in the back of the neck because of the weakness that can be associated with those injections.

I think that the perceived weakness of the neck following injections with botulinum toxin is not due to the neck muscles indeed being weak, because the amount of toxin injected in them is too small. It is more, I think, because the muscles in the back of the neck tighten further due to the irritation caused by the injections. This irritation further increases the resting tone of the muscles and that, in turn, makes them feel weak. Either way, it does not help the patient feel any better when it happens, and we can avoid it altogether by omitting the injections in the back of the neck.

Apart from treating the neck muscle tightness, preferably with daily heat from a microwavable heating pad administered twice daily for fifteen to twenty minutes, we need to treat the headaches resulting from it, and we should do so with medications. Of course, we can also use physical therapy modalities other than daily heat to treat the neck muscle tightness; as far as I am concerned, however, daily heat should be the basis of the treatment.

With the daily heat, it is important that we apply the heating pad relatively low to cover not only the neck but also the shoulders and upper back. It is equally important to keep the heat away from the head, because especially when the headaches have a migraine quality, heat transmitted to the head will make them worse, which of course we do not want.

If we prescribe physical therapy to help resolve the neck muscle tightness, it is important that the therapist has experience treating headache patients and treats the muscles gently not to aggravate the headaches. Sending them to random therapists, in my experience, results in about half of the patients coming back, reporting worsening of their headaches. Consequently, I have become reluctant to send them to therapists I do not know or with whom I have not already had good experience.

For neck-related problems, I prefer passive modalities, like heat, ultrasound, and gentle massage. This is different with low back pain, for which I prefer active modalities, such as stretching and strengthening. The active modalities, in my experience, are too harsh for the neck muscles and tend to make matters worse.

Medications

With regard to medication treatment, we do not have specific medications for chronic post-traumatic headache, which is what we call it when headaches persist following a head or neck injury. Instead, we base our treatment on the presentation of the headaches, and we generally diagnose them as migraine when they are intense.

Due to the association with tight neck, shoulder, upper back, and often, also jaw muscles, the headache frequency is generally high. This means that in terms of presentation, we are most likely dealing here with high-frequency episodic migraine or chronic migraine.

Regardless of the presentation, the patient needs effective abortive treatment that fully relieves the headaches within two hours, consistently and without side effects. Allowing them to continue to suffer repeatedly from headaches, especially when intense, will over time set them back and worsen their condition.

In general, we provide abortive migraine treatment most effectively with specific medications; at present, these are the triptans and gepants. We have seven triptans that we can prescribe, including one that we can administer by subcutaneous injection for fast and powerful relief, as well as three gepants. The seven triptans are almotriptan, eletriptan, frovatriptan, naratriptan, rizatriptan, sumatriptan, and zolmitriptan, of which sumatriptan is the one that we can give by injection as well. The three gepants for abortive treatment are rimegepant, ubrogepant, and zavegepant.

For preventive migraine treatment, we have four CGRP antibodies and two gepants. We should certainly apply preventive treatment in chronic post-traumatic headache, in addition to effective abortive treatment, given the generally high frequency of the headaches. The four CGRP antibodies are eptinezumab, erenumab, fremanezumab, and galcanezumab; the two gepants for preventive treatment are atogepant and rimegepant.

In the absence of intense headaches and with a presentation resembling chronic tension headache, we can employ a relatively small dose of a tricyclic, like imipramine or nortriptyline, for preventive treatment.

If we use a muscle relaxant, I prefer the fast- and short-acting ones abortively for mild headaches, such as metaxalone or carisoprodol. The dose of metaxalone is 800 milligrams, and that of carisoprodol is 350 milligrams; patients can take them as needed for headache every four to six hours. They generally tolerate the metaxalone well, without side effects, while carisoprodol sometimes causes drowsiness.

In general, I avoid the long-acting muscle relaxants, such as cyclobenzaprine or tizanidine, which we prescribe once daily at bedtime, because they often cause daytime drowsiness or fatigue. I have found that patients generally tolerate the tricyclics, which they also take once daily at bedtime, better and find them more effective as well, the latter probably because they combine muscle relaxant and pain relieving, or analgesic, benefits.

Concussion Syndrome

Experimental studies in rodents have shown that a whiplash injury of the neck can unleash the sympathetic nervous system, resulting in symptoms that affect the body as a whole. As discussed earlier, the sympathetic nervous system is the part of the involuntary or autonomic nervous system activated by mental or physical stress;

its activation makes our heart pound and gives us butterflies in the stomach.

It also increases our heart rate, which makes us feel on edge or even anxious, and heightens our level of arousal, which can render us anxious as well and, in addition, may affect our ability to concentrate. This, in turn, can cause problems storing and retrieving memory and potentially impairs our cognitive functioning, making us feel like in a brain fog. Finally, it may render us irritable; as a result, we can have problems sleeping at night. We may also feel short of breath and develop issues with nausea or constipation.

Armed with this knowledge, we can try to reign in the unleashed sympathetic nervous system, in addition to treating the individual complaints of what we call concussion syndrome. We can attempt to do so with relaxation techniques, of which a great variety is available, or with a medication called clonidine.

This medication has been on the market since the 1960s for the treatment of hypertension and for that of attention deficit and hyperactivity disorder, or ADHD, in children, teenagers, and adolescents. We also employ it for the treatment of anxiety and menopausal night sweats or hot flashes, and it can be beneficial as well mitigating the symptoms of nicotine or opioid withdrawal.

We generally prescribe it in a dose of 0.1 milligram once or twice daily, and if indicated and the patient tolerates it well, we can also use higher dosages. The most common side effects of clonidine are drowsiness and dry mouth; it does not have contraindications. The medication is also available in a skin patch for weekly application, preferred by some over taking a tablet daily.

Chapter 16

What about the Pain in My Face?

Face Pain

Although the face is part of the head, face pain is a very different problem from headaches. It is also quite common, although not as common as headaches, and affects approximately 7 percent of the population. In comparison, irritable bowel syndrome impacts approximately the same proportion of the population, and so does chronic fatigue. Migraine, on the other hand, is twice as common and affects approximately 15 percent of the population.

The burden for society that face pain presents is, however, not as great as that of headaches, if only because the intensity of the pain does not tend to be as high. This does not mean to say that face pain cannot be intense or even excruciatingly so and life-changing, because it can. However, at least in my experience, this is less often the case than with headaches.

An interesting observation is that face pain is more commonly associated with headaches, including migraine, than the other way around, at least in medical practice. This may solely be because patients with face pain are more likely to seek medical consultation, if headaches trouble them as well. After all, there is undoubtedly a limit as to how much pain people can tolerate in their lives.

Another explanation could be that the mechanism behind face pain is often muscular which, similarly to neck muscle tightness, drives headache frequency. This results in headaches occurring frequently, daily or almost daily, which also prompts medical consultation, although by far not to the extent that headache intensity does.

The primary driver of medical consultation for headache is, in my experience, headache intensity, not headache frequency. Generally, people do not seek medical intervention for headaches that they can easily treat themselves—for example, with nonprescription pain medications—even when they happen frequently.

Diagnosis

We diagnose face pain differently from the so-called primary headache conditions, such as tension headache, migraine, cluster headache, and stabbing headache. These disorders, which account for the vast majority of headache suffering in the world, we diagnose based on the intensity of the headaches and their temporal pattern.

We generally divide headache intensity into three categories—mild, moderate, and severe—depending on the extent to which they affect the ability to function physically. If they do not impact the physical ability to function, we call them mild; if they do affect the ability to function but not in a way that they require bed rest, we refer to them as moderate; if the headaches are so intense that they necessitate bed rest, even for a short period, we call them severe.

When talking about temporal pattern, I am referring to how the headaches occur over time. For example, do they happen in attacks, called paroxysms? Alternatively, are they present more or less all the time, meaning daily and continuously or more or less so?

When the headaches are paroxysmal and occur in attacks, it is important to know how long they last in terms of days, hours, minutes, or seconds. In this way, we diagnose headaches that are mild and happen in attacks as episodic tension headache and when they are continuous or more or less so as chronic tension headache.

If attacks of moderate or severe headache last a good part of a day or days, we diagnose them as migraine; if they last one to two hours, as cluster headache. We diagnose the headaches as paroxysmal hemicrania if they last ten to thirty minutes and as stabbing headache if they last seconds.

If the moderate or severe headaches are non-paroxysmal and are present daily and continuously or more or less so, we diagnose them as chronic migraine. We diagnose the so-called secondary headache conditions, in which medical or neurological illness causes the headaches, based on the findings on physical examination and additional testing, such as blood tests or imaging.

Trigeminal Neuralgia

As mentioned, we diagnose face pain differently from headaches and do so based on its location in the face and its presentation as jabbing, stabbing, or lancinating, on the one hand, or continuous, on the other.

The face pain disorder undoubtedly best known to physicians and other health care practitioners is trigeminal neuralgia, a disabling condition with intense jabbing pain in the face that hits like lightning and lasts seconds. It is rare, however, and probably as uncommon as cluster headache, which is an equally devastating pain disorder.

The pain occurs on the right or left side of the face only, never on both sides, and never switches sides, akin to the headaches of cluster headache. At the same time, it never affects the entire half of the face but always just part of it, depending on which branch of the trigeminal nerve is impacted.

The latter is the nerve that provides sensation to the face with the first, or ophthalmic, branch going to the forehead; the second, or maxillary, branch going to the cheek; and the third, or mandibular, branch going to the jaw. Most commonly involved is the branch to the cheek, which is the maxillary branch, followed by the branch to the jaw, the mandibular branch, and occasionally both.

Rarely does the condition affect the forehead, or ophthalmic branch, but here we may experience the pain from stabbing headache, which is very similar to that of trigeminal neuralgia but of a different origin. Consequently, the treatment is different, because trigeminal neuralgia is nerve related while stabbing headache is migraine related. As a migraine-related disorder, it can occur in any part of the face and is not limited to particular areas, as trigeminal neuralgia is.

Neuropathic Pain

In medicine, we refer to nerve pain as neuropathic pain and often base its diagnosis on the quality of the pain as jabbing, stabbing, or lancinating, on the one hand, or burning, on the other. However, as far as I am concerned, neither description is diagnostic of neuropathic pain in the same way as itching is not diagnostic of a skin reaction being allergic, because it can also be inflammatory.

As we have seen, jabbing pain in the face does not have to be nerve related, or neuropathic, but can also be migraine related, as in stabbing headache. Of course, when it occurs in the face, we should call it stabbing face pain instead, because it is face pain rather than headache.

Nerve damage causes neuropathic pain, and in trigeminal neuralgia, supposedly, a blood vessel pressing on the trigeminal ganglion damages the nerve. The trigeminal ganglion is the nerve knot at the base of the brain from which the three branches of the trigeminal nerve originate.

A diagnosis of nerve pain requires indications of nerve damage, which imply that the nerve is not working well. As the trigeminal nerve is a sensory nerve that provides feeling to the face, such indications would be an abnormal processing of sensory information coming from the face.

We generally test this by gently touching the face in its three divisions—the forehead, cheek, and jaw—and note how the patient responds to the touch. With damage to the nerve, they may feel it as tingling, which we call paresthesia. If it feels unpleasant—for example, as if touched with a cold rod—we call it dysesthesia. If they actually feel the touch as pain or if it provokes a painful jab in the face, as is typical in trigeminal neuralgia, we call it allodynia.

The presence of allodynia is highly characteristic of trigeminal neuralgia, and subtly touching the face, like by a gentle breeze, can provoke the jabbing pain. Such indications of nerve damage are, of course, not present in the migraine-related stabbing face pain because of its different origin.

However, nerve pain does not have to be stabbing; in fact, it is not in the majority of cases and wherever located in the body. Most of the time, it is continuous, as in the unrelenting foot pain that diabetics may suffer from, called diabetic painful neuropathy, or DPN.

In my experience, diabetics with nerve foot pain describe their pain as burning, like fire or hot coal, as frequently as they relate to it as numbness, which can be burning or tingling. They also often describe it as tingling numbness or pins and needles, or mention razor blade sharp pain, cramping, throbbing, or heaviness. In other words, a whole series of adjectives can be associated with neuropathic pain, not just *stabbing* or *burning*.

Neuropathic Face Pain

If neuropathic pain in the face is continuous, with or without superimposed jabbing, stabbing, or lancinating pain, we call it painful trigeminal neuropathy. In this condition, the pain is always located just on the right or left side of the face and limited to one of the three divisions of the trigeminal nerve: the forehead, cheek, or jaw.

In addition to the persistent pain, however described, evidence of nerve damage must be present to call it neuropathic. Such evidence can be paresthesia, tingling on gentle touch; dysesthesia, an unpleasant sensation on gentle touch; or allodynia, pain on gentle touch.

An example of painful trigeminal neuropathy is ophthalmic zoster, also called zoster ophthalmicus, a form of herpes zoster or shingles. It affects the ophthalmic branch of the trigeminal nerve and causes pain in the right or left side of the forehead, in contrast to the usual presentation of herpes zoster, which causes pain in the right or left side of the trunk.

Herpes zoster is quite common in people over sixty, but fortunately, it rarely strikes the face. However, when it does, it is very painful, and I have seen it in the mouth as well where, as you can imagine, it makes eating a living hell.

Little blisters appear several days after the onset of the pain, usually in small groups. They may be very obvious and easy to see, but they can also be hard to find and may require some looking around. In ophthalmic zoster, they can be hiding in the hairline, or one or two may be present between the eyelashes.

We should consider ophthalmic zoster in every older patient reporting pain in one side of the forehead that started recently, within days or a week or so. We should carefully search for the little blisters, or scabs if they are healing, to confirm the diagnosis and initiate treatment as soon as possible.

The treatment consists of an antiviral medication, like acyclovir or valacyclovir, started within seventy-two hours of the onset of symptoms, if possible. As mentioned, pain is usually the initial complaint, but it does not have to be; it can be itching or tingling instead.

The pain, when present, is often intense, and we should combine the antiviral medication with pain treatment, as appropriate. In addition, the patient should see an eye specialist, or ophthalmologist, because the condition, through scarring of the cornea, can also affect vision and potentially cause blindness.

Continuous Face Pain

If the pain in the face is not jabbing, stabbing, or lancinating and there is no indication that it is due to nerve damage, it tends to be present continuously. Of course, other paroxysmal presentations than stabbing are possible as well, but they are rare.

Occasionally, migraine causes pain in the face; if it does, as in facial migraine, the pain is present for a day or so and is associated with nausea and, sometimes, also with vomiting. More likely than with migraine, the pain of cluster headache can be situated in the face, for example in the cheek, lasting one to two hours at a time.

With continuous pain in the face that is not due to nerve damage, location is key in determining the diagnosis. It has two aspects: right or left or on both sides—that is, unilateral or bilateral—and central or peripheral. The latter describes whether the pain is predominantly situated in the nose-cheek area, centrally in the face, or in the jaw or jaws, peripherally in the face.

Peripheral face pain that is not due to nerve damage originates from the jaw muscles that we call masseter muscles. We have four pairs of jaw muscles, the so-called muscles of mastication, of which three close the mouth and one opens it.

The masseter muscles comprise one of the three pairs that close the mouth; the other two pairs are the medial pterygoid muscles and the temporalis muscles. The remaining pair of the four pairs of jaw, or masticatory, muscles is that of the lateral pterygoid muscles which, aided by gravity, open the mouth.

In so-called temporomandibular disorder, or TMD, the muscles of mastication do not function properly; they are tight and painful, causing pain in the jaw or jaws in the area on the outside of the face, where we can feel the masseter muscle. If the jaw pain is on both sides, it tends to be low-grade, often merely described as a discomfort or ache. I like to refer to it as masseter tension or call it the facial variant of chronic tension headache.

It is different when the pain is on one side only, or unilateral. Then it is likely intense, sometimes associated with stabbing or with visible twitching of the affected muscle. If this is the case, I refer to it as masseter spasm, a condition that can be confusing because it can cause so-called referred pain in the upper or lower teeth in the back of the mouth, the molars. These teeth hurt not because something is wrong with them but due to the spasm of the adjacent masseter muscle.

As temporomandibular disorder is sometimes associated with stabbing pain in the jaw area, we may confuse it with trigeminal neuralgia. However, here the stabbing occurs on a background of continuous pain, which is not the case in trigeminal neuralgia; in addition, no indications of nerve damage are present. In particular, we cannot provoke the pain by gently touching the face, although we may be able to do so by palpating the affected masseter muscle, but that, of course, is not the same.

Central Face Pain

When the pain is located centrally in the face, which means in the nose-cheek area, we are dealing with a nose-sinus problem. Like the jaw pain, it tends to be low-grade when bilateral and located on both sides or high-grade when unilateral and limited to the right or left side only.

When on both sides, patients often describe it as a pressure rather than a pain, like a plunger stuck on the face or a mask pulled tightly to the back. Underpressure in the sinuses causes this drawing sensation centrally in the face, which is a condition that we refer to as sinus vacuum or barosinusitis.

The colloquial term is sinus headache, but this is a misnomer, because it is much more a cause of face pain than of headache. The center of the forehead and the bridge of the nose may be the predominant site of the discomfort or pain, if it mostly involves the frontal sinuses.

The underlying problem is blockage of the openings through which the sinuses communicate with the outside world, which can be narrow from birth, or congenitally. When this is indeed the case, even mild nasal congestion, as due to allergies or nasal irritation, can close them off. Exposure to secondhand smoke or to a strong odor or smell, even when pleasant, can be the source of such irritation.

As the air in the closed-off sinuses gets absorbed, underpressure develops and, consequently, the drawing feeling in the center of the face. In a migraineur, this sensation often quickly evolves into a migraine headache, resulting in a "bad sinus headache." However, the intense pain does not originate from the sinuses but from a genetically determined and inherited migraine vulnerability. Hence, we should treat it as such and not as a sinus problem, which it is not, although the trigger resides in the nose.

It is a very different story when the central face pain is unilateral and limited to one side of the face only; then the pain can be so intense that it is life-changing. Hard intranasal contact is often the culprit, easily recognizable if you think of it, simple to diagnose with computerized tomography of the nose and sinuses, and easily treated by an ear-nose-and-throat (ENT) surgeon, or otolaryngologist.

The intranasal contact is hard in the sense that it is bony, caused by a spur, or spina, coming off a deviated septum and, like a splinter, driving into the side of the nose. The pain is usually of acute onset due to congestion of the nose from a head cold or flu or from a flare-up of allergies, with the congestion creating the contact, subsequently maintained by a vicious inflammatory cycle.

I once saw the contact established during an emotional outburst, accompanied by crying and, consequently, by nasal congestion. The outburst was caused by a robbery, resulting in a psychological interpretation of the persistent, severe face pain that followed. When psychotherapy did not provide benefit, a neurologist diagnosed the patient with cluster headache because of the association of the pain with tearing and congestion.

When his treatment did not relieve the pain either, I saw the patient and diagnosed her with intranasal contact based on the face pain presentation. I confirmed the diagnosis with computerized tomography of the nose and sinuses and provided her with temporary solace using lidocaine nose drops. I referred her to an ear-nose-and-throat surgeon, who eliminated the spur, ending years of suffering.

She subsequently became pregnant, which she had postponed because she did not consider herself capable of caring for a child while struggling with the pain.

Treatment

Not only is the diagnosis of face pain very different from that of headaches, the treatment is very different as well. For me, when it comes to medications, botulinum toxin plays a greater role in the treatment of face pain than in that of headaches, where we use it for chronic migraine.

In chronic migraine, we administer 155 units in total and do so over thirty-one injections in the forehead, temples, back of the head, back of the neck, and shoulders and repeat it, if beneficial, every three months. In face pain, I use the toxin in particular for the treatment of trigeminal neuralgia, as well as for pain originating from the masseter muscle or muscles.

In medicine, we generally treat trigeminal neuralgia with medications like carbamazepine and oxcarbazepine, both originally anti-epilepsy medications, also called anti-seizure medications or anticonvulsants. We employ the latter extensively for the treatment of chronic pain, including headaches, particularly if the pain is due to nerve damage—that is, when neuropathic.

Trigeminal neuralgia is a form of neuropathic pain, and we consider carbamazepine and oxcarbazepine the medications of choice to treat it. We generally prescribe them two times per day—carbamazepine starting at one hundred milligrams twice daily and oxcarbazepine at three hundred milligrams twice daily. We subsequently slowly increase the dose called uptitration, until we obtain good pain relief, but patients often do not tolerate the medications well because of side effects, especially carbamazepine.

Common side effects of those anticonvulsants are dizziness, drowsiness, impaired balance, fatigue, and vertigo. Especially in older patients, who are the ones who develop trigeminal neuralgia, such side effects can be disastrous, because they lead to falls and fractures.

Consequently, I prefer to treat these patients with botulinum toxin, which has the advantage of good tolerability with few, if any, side effects. With a tiny needle, I inject small amounts of the toxin into the affected skin and, if involved in the pain as well, into the gum. I generally also inject it into the masseter muscle on the side of the pain, palpating for taut bands.

For neuropathic pain that is present continuously, such as in ophthalmic zoster, we usually prescribe anticonvulsants that patients generally tolerate better. These medications are gabapentin and pregabalin, which belong to the class of gabapentinoids, medications derived from a naturally occurring chemical in the brain called gamma-aminobutyric acid, or GABA. A substance of abuse, gamma-hydroxybutyric acid, or GHB, is a derivative of the same chemical; possibly related to that, gabapentin and pregabalin are so-called controlled substances but scheduled in the class with the lowest risk of abuse.

We generally prescribe gabapentin and pregabalin in three divided dosages over the day, approximately eight hours apart. They can cause drowsiness and dizziness and may impair balance as well. Therefore, we should always start with a low dose, such as 100 milligrams of gabapentin or 25 milligrams of pregabalin thrice daily. We can increase these dosages with weekly intervals but should do so slowly, carefully monitoring tolerability.

The fact that both are available in numerous dose strengths makes this slow uptitration relatively easy. Gabapentin is available in dosages ranging from 100 to 800 milligrams per tablet, and pregabalin in those ranging from 25 to 300 milligrams per tablet. The maximum daily dose for gabapentin is 3,600 milligrams, and that for pregabalin is 600 milligrams.

Indomethacin

Stabbing face pain, the facial equivalent of stabbing headache, we treat with indomethacin, provided the frequency of the pain justifies such an aggressive approach. It is a potent medication to treat headache and pain, but it also potently upsets the stomach. Therefore, it should always be taken with food and probably also always with a medication to protect the stomach, such as a proton-pump inhibitor, or PPI.

The initial dose is usually twenty-five milligrams four times per day with the meals and at bedtime or seventy-five milligrams, sustained release, at breakfast and twenty-five milligrams at bedtime. If we omit the bedtime dose with either regimen, withdrawal headache develops overnight, resulting in a dull, throbbing pain in the back of the head on awakening in the morning. If necessary, we can increase the dose to seventy-five milligrams, sustained release, twice daily at breakfast and at dinner or fifty milligrams four times per day with the meals and at bedtime.

With long-term use of the medication, it is important to monitor kidney function and follow the patient carefully for the development of gastritis, which is inflammation of the lining of the stomach. Complaints like nausea, heartburn, acid reflux, or stomach pain can develop but may not be prominent or can even be absent.

Gastritis caused by nonsteroidal anti-inflammatory drugs, or NSAIDs, such as indomethacin, can be completely without symptoms, or asymptomatic. The only manifestation may be the development of anemia due to chronic blood loss in the stool, which is occult and, hence, not visible to the naked eye because it is minimal. However, it adds up over time and can cause a significant drop in hemoglobin and iron reserve, or ferritin. The insidious development of fatigue due to iron-deficiency anemia may be the only indication that something is amiss.

Muscles

Pain in the jaw on one or both sides requires a muscular approach, particularly directed at the muscles that close the mouth. Of these, we can feel the masseter muscles in the outside of the jaws and the temporalis muscles in the temples. In general, it is difficult to get tight muscles to relax, however, and for our efforts to be successful, we may need to apply several approaches at the same time.

A vicious cycle may be present with the tight muscles squeezing off their circulation, consequently depriving themselves of oxygen for efficient energy metabolism, on the one hand, and of effective elimination of waste products, on the other. In case of the jaw-closing muscles, they may additionally find themselves caught in a cycle of bruxism—in other words, clenching and grinding.

Tight jaw muscles cause the abnormal functional activities of clenching and grinding, which in turn make them tighter. In order to interrupt this vicious cycle, there may be an indication for appliance therapy with a mouth guard, also called occlusal splint or orthotic device. We employ mouth guards in two ways depending on whether we place them on the lower teeth or on the upper teeth.

The lower-teeth mouth guard, or mandibular device, we usually wear when we are up and about during the day. The upper-teeth mouth guard, or maxillary device, on the other hand, we wear during sleep which is generally at night but can also be during the day. Both types serve the purpose of preventing clenching and grinding, and equally important, they protect the teeth from the wear caused by these so-called parafunctional activities.

Additionally helpful is the daily use of heat on the muscles for fifteen to twenty minutes each time, preferably with a microwavable heating pad. We can combine this daily heat application with gentle stretching of the jaw muscles by carefully opening the mouth widely. Formal physical therapy in the form of massage and ultrasound may be effective as well, along with techniques like acupressure or acupuncture.

We can also utilize injection treatment, either in the form of so-called trigger point injections with a local anesthetic, like lidocaine, or injections with botulinum toxin. I prefer the latter for the masseter muscles because of its much longer-lasting benefit and administer twenty-five to thirty-five units of the toxin in each muscle. With either injection technique and although I do not know whether it makes a difference, I target the taut bands that I can palpate in the muscles.

Patients generally tolerate the injections well, and even when I perform them with botulinum toxin, they do not affect jaw closure. This is undoubtedly because of the excess muscular reserve that is present in closing the mouth, with three pairs of muscles involved.

Nose

Face pain of central location, affecting the nose, cheek or cheeks, and center of the forehead, we treat depending on the cause. With pain on both sides, chronic allergic rhinitis is often the culprit, which we treat with an anti-allergy nasal spray. For this purpose, we can use an antihistamine nasal spray, such as azelastine, a mast cell-stabilizing nasal spray, such as cromolyn, or a corticosteroid, or steroid, nasal spray.

For best result, I always recommend administering the azelastine or cromolyn nasal spray four times per day. The corticosteroid nasal sprays we can effectively use twice daily, and several of them are available, prescription and nonprescription, including budesonide, fluticasone, and triamcinolone.

In general, I think that patients tolerate the water-based corticosteroid nasal sprays better than the alcohol-based ones, especially with long-term use. This is particularly the case when it comes to dryness of the nose and nosebleeds as potential side effects. We recognize the water-based nasal sprays by the inclusion of *Aqua* or *AQ* in the brand name.

Intranasal contact is often the cause of central face pain that is unilateral and limited to one side of the face only, right or left. As this is hard or bony contact, it requires surgical intervention in the form of a minimally corrective endoscopic procedure. An experienced ear-nose-and-throat, or ENT, surgeon should perform it, consisting of elimination of the contact.

The intranasal contact generally originates from a spur, called spina, coming off a deviated septum, which the surgeon should correct as well to prevent recurrence. Otherwise, they should not remove anything from the nose, including the impacted swell body on the side of the nose, called turbinate.

Swell bodies, or turbinates, are important structures in the nose to warm up and moisturize the inhaled air. In the same vein, they should leave the sinuses alone and definitely not open them up excessively. Wide-open communications from the nose to the sinuses cause sensitivity problems, which may ultimately make breathing through the nose uncomfortable, if not painful.

In case of intranasal contact, decongestant nasal sprays, which shrink the lining of the nose, and corticosteroid nasal sprays, which reduce the associated inflammation, can be helpful as well. In addition, a local anesthetic, like lidocaine, applied to the inside of the nose at the site of the contact can provide immediate relief. Such positive effect definitely increases the likelihood that surgical intervention will have the desired benefit, but lack thereof surely does not preclude it.

I have rarely seen one-sided, or unilateral, central face pain caused by a dental problem, but it is certainly possible. Then the culprit is one of the front teeth in the upper jaw, called maxillary incisors. They can cause pain in the side of the nose or in the cheek depending on whether the inner, central, or outer, lateral, incisor is affected.

The problem can be in the tooth itself, like an infection, which may ultimately require a root canal procedure, but it can also be in the ligament. The latter keeps the tooth fixed in the jaw socket and, like a tendon, can become inflamed. We treat such an inflammation, like a tendinitis, with a nonsteroidal anti-inflammatory drug, or NSAID. Of course, with either condition, a dentist can extract the tooth; obviously, that is not the preferred treatment. Preferred treatments always preserve structure and function.

Acknowledgments

First and foremost, I would like to thank my mentor, John R. Graham, who took me under his wing when I was a medical student, introduced me to headache, and taught me all he knew. Spiritually, he connected me with his mentor, Harold G. Wolff, for whom he had great respect and admiration.

In addition to the factual knowledge that Professor Graham passed on to me about headache and medicine, he taught me to listen to patients. I consider this his greatest gift, because it allowed me to continue my learning from the ones who are the experiential experts, namely, those afflicted by headache. From the headache sufferers whom I saw as patients, I gained the most, and I am grateful to them for allowing me to learn from them while involved in their care.

Second, I would like to thank the many colleagues whom I had the pleasure and privilege collaborating with to the benefit of my patients and learning from them in the process. Particularly, I would like to mention the endocrinologist and thyroid specialist, the late Kenneth R. Blanchard; the psychiatrist and psychopharmacologist Eric C. Dessain; the otolaryngologist Harsha V. Gopal; the optometrist Ernest V. Loewenstein; the dentist and craniofacial pain specialist Noshir R. Mehta; and the hematologist and oncologist, the late James A. Warth.

Third, I would like to thank my wife, Maria K. B. Spierings-Zarska, MA, Stacey J. Miller, MA, and the copyediting team of Fulton Books for assistance in the preparation of the manuscript, and my friend and colleague Padma J. Narayan, PhD, for critically reviewing Chapter 7.

Fourth, I would like to thank my family, friends, and everyone dear to me for tolerating my obsession with headache in addition to working long hours. It was not until I got diagnosed with kidney cancer in 2015 that I realized that there is more to life than work. I am grateful for this realization and the opportunity it provided me to return to my old and cherished hobbies: playing the guitar and horseback riding.

Fifth, I would like to thank my colleagues and coworkers at Boston Advanced Medicine, formerly Boston PainCare, for welcoming me to their family. Families like that are precious, and you can never have enough of them.

Glossary

akathisia: Restlessness
algometer: Device to measure pain threshold
allodynia: Pain caused by an ordinarily painless stimulus
amaurosis fugax: Temporary blindness of one eye
anemia: Low hemoglobin
aneurysm: Localized expansion of an artery like a little balloon
angina: Chest pain from temporary blockage of blood flow to part of the heart
arteriovenous malformation: Congenital blood vessel abnormality
benign intracranial hypertension: Increased pressure in the head due to swelling of the brain
bruxism: Clenching and grinding
cerebral: Related to the brain
cerebral circulation: Brain blood flow
cerebrum: Brain
cerebellum: Small brain located in the back of the head
cerebrospinal fluid: Fluid present in and around the brain and spinal cord
cheiro-oral syndrome: Tingling generally commencing in the fingers of one hand, gradually moving up the arm, and ultimately involving the nose-mouth area
ciliary muscle: Muscle in the eye that surrounds the lens
cobalamin: Vitamin B_{12}
comorbidity: Accompanying medical condition
conjunctival injection: Reddening of the eye
digitolingual paresthesias: *See* cheiro-oral syndrome
dolometer: *See* algometer
dysesthesia: Unpleasant sensation upon gently touching the skin
dysmenorrhea: Painful menstruation

dura mater: Outer membrane of the brain attached to the inside of the skull
eclampsia: Hypertension-related seizures during pregnancy
encephalitis: Inflammation of the brain
encephalopathy: Brain disease
epidural hematoma: Bleeding between the dura mater and the skull
epigastric area: Stomach area of the abdomen
extracranial: Outside the skull
fibromyalgia: Muscle soreness or pain affecting trunk and extremities
fortification spectra: *See* scintillating scotoma
frontotemporal area: Area between forehead and temple
gangrene: Tissue death
gastritis: Inflammation of the lining of the stomach
gastrocolic reflex: Reflex connecting the stomach with the large bowel
glabella: Area of skin between the eyebrows
giant cell arteritis: Inflammation of the arteries of the body, including the head
Hashimoto's thyroiditis: Autoimmune thyroid disease
histaminic cephalalgia: Cluster headache
Horton's headache: Cluster headache
hydrocephalus: Enlargement of the chambers in the brain and brain stem
hypermenorrhea: Long or heavy menstruation
hypersomnolence: Sleeping excessively, including prolonged napping during the day
hypertension: High blood pressure
hyperthyroidism: High thyroid function; overactive thyroid
hypothyroidism: Low thyroid function; underactive thyroid
intramuscularly: In a muscle
intravenously: In a vein
lacrimation: Tearing of the eye
lumbago: Low back pain
lymphatic system: System that brings tissue fluid back into the blood
mandibular nerve: Branch of the trigeminal nerve providing sensation to the jaw

maxillary nerve: Branch of the trigeminal nerve providing sensation to the cheek
menarche: First occurrence of menstruation
meningioma: Benign tumor originating from the dura mater
meningitis: Inflammation of the two inner membranes of the brain
menorrhagia: *See* hypermenorrhea
metrorrhagia: Long or heavy vaginal bleeding unrelated to menstruation
migrainous neuralgia: Cluster headache
miosis: Small pupil
neuropathy: Nerve disease
nociceptive: Related to pain perception
odorphobia: Heightened sensitivity to smell
oligomenorrhea: Menstruation occurring less often than monthly
ophthalmic nerve: Branch of the trigeminal nerve providing sensation to the forehead
ophthalmic zoster: Shingles affecting the sensory nerve to the forehead
osmophobia: Heightened sensitivity to smell
paradoxical diarrhea: Diarrhea caused by constipation
paresthesia: Tingling sensation upon gently touching the skin
paroxysm: Attack
paroxysmal: Occurring in attacks
perimenstrually: Around the time of menstruation
peristalsis: Forward movement of stomach and bowel
phonophobia: Heightened sensitivity to sound
photophobia: Heightened sensitivity to light
polymenorrhea: Menstruation occurring more often than monthly
pseudotumor cerebri: *See* benign intracranial hypertension
ptosis: Drooping of the upper eyelid
puerperium: Six-week period following delivery
pulsation amplitude: Magnitude of the throbbing of an artery
rhinorrhea: Running of the nose
scintillating scotoma: Crescent or half-moon of flickering, zigzag lines
soma: Body
subarachnoid hemorrhage: Bleeding between the two inner membranes of the brain

subcutaneously: Under the skin
subdural hematoma: Bleeding between the two outer membranes of the brain
superficial temporal artery: Artery that runs from the temple to the forehead
temporal arteritis: *See* giant cell arteritis
teichopsia: *See* scintillating scotoma
thyroiditis: Inflammation of the thyroid gland
transient ischemic attack: Mini stroke or mini brain attack
trigeminal ganglion: Nerve knot at the base of the brain from which the trigeminal nerve originates
trigeminal nerve: Nerve originating from the trigeminal ganglion providing sensation to the face
uptitration: Gradually increasing the dose of a medication
vasoconstriction: Narrowing of blood vessels
vasodilation: Widening of blood vessels
ventricular system: System of chambers in the brain and brain stem
vertex: Top of the head

About the Author

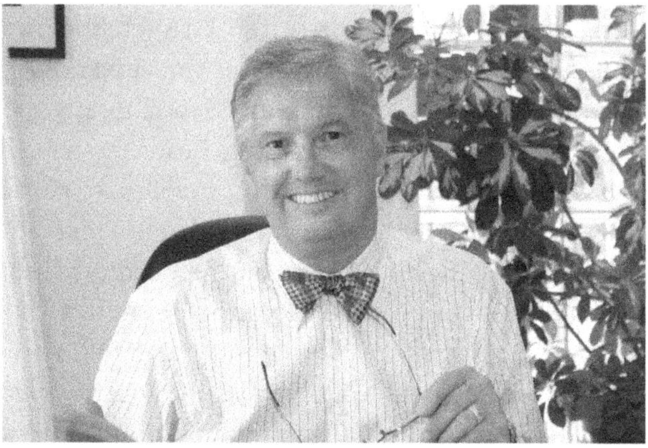

Dr. Spierings is a pharmacologist, neurologist, headache and face pain specialist, and clinical trialist. He was born in Helmond, the Netherlands, in 1953. He attended the Erasmus University Faculty of Medicine in Rotterdam, the Netherlands, where he received a bachelor's degree in medical sciences in 1974, a master's degree in medical sciences in 1976, a medical doctor degree in 1978, and a doctor of philosophy degree in experimental pharmacology in 1980.

In terms of postgraduate education, he trained in neurosurgery (1980–1981) and neurology (1982–1984) at the University Hospital Dijkzigt, now Erasmus Medical Center, in Rotterdam, the Netherlands; in psychiatry (1985) at the Reinier de Graaf Gasthuis in Delft, the oldest hospital in the Netherlands; and in headache management (1981–1982) at the Headache Research Foundation at Faulkner Hospital in Boston, Massachusetts.

He became the director of the Headache Research Foundation at Faulkner Hospital in 1986, succeeding his headache mentor, John R. Graham, MD, MACP. He established the John R. Graham Headache

Center at Faulkner Hospital in 1987 and moved to Brigham and Women's Hospital and Harvard Medical School in 1990.

He was an associate professor of neurology, part-time academic faculty, at Harvard Medical School from 1999 until 2014 and a professor of neurology and craniofacial pain, part-time academic faculty, at Tufts University Schools of Medicine and Dental Medicine from 2014 until 2018, when he retired from academia. Since 2019, he has been the medical director of the Greater Boston Headache Center and MedVadis Research at Boston Advanced Medicine, formerly Boston PainCare, in Waltham, Massachusetts.

Dr. Spierings has been conducting headache-related research since he was a medical student, that is, for almost half a century. He has been involved in headache management since he became a neurologist in 1985 with his practice entirely dedicated to headache and face pain. For over almost four decades, he has treated thousands of patients, most of them with migraine, and followed them for years, if not decades. At one time, he was the fourth biggest triptan prescriber in the United States and, thus, probably in the world.

Based on his extensive clinical experience, Dr. Spierings described hemicrania continua as an indomethacin-responsive headache syndrome, developed the high-dose verapamil treatment for cluster headache, and conceptualized the parallel theory of migraine pathogenesis. More recently, his interest has been the comorbidities of chronic migraine, for which he coined the term systemic endocrine-metabolic syndrome, or SEMS.

He has lectured extensively in North and South America, Europe, and Australia and has organized twenty-six symposia at Harvard Medical School and Tufts University Schools of Medicine and Dental Medicine, among others. He has authored, coauthored, or edited more than three hundred publications, including the following books:

- *De Pathogenese van Migraine* (Stafleu's Scientific Publishing Company, Alphen aan den Rijn, the Netherlands, 1982)
- *Hoofdpijn* (Scientific Publishing Company Bunge, Utrecht, the Netherlands, 1984)

- *Migraine* (Sandoz Pharmaceuticals, Basel, Switzerland, 1986)
- *Migraine: Questions and Answers* (Merit Publishing International, West Palm Beach, Florida, 1995 and 2002)
- *Management of Migraine* (Butterworth-Heinemann, Boston, Massachusetts, 1996; Japanese translation published by Shidan-To-Chiryosha Company, 1997)
- *Headache* (Butterworth-Heinemann, Boston, Massachusetts, 1998)
- *Migraine Diagnostiek & Therapie* (Cure & Care Publishers, Zeist, the Netherlands, 2001)
- *Migraine: A Neuroinflammatory Disease?* (Birkhäuser Verlag, Basel, Switzerland, 2002)

He is also the section editor on headache and pain of the textbook *Office Practice of Neurology*, edited by Martin A. Samuels and Steven K. Feske (Churchill Livingstone, Philadelphia, Pennsylvania, 1996 and 2003).

Dr. Spierings has a son, Sven E. J. Spierings, who is a design architect, entrepreneur, and application developer (Tapsody.com) and lives in Rotterdam, the Netherlands. He also has a daughter, Natalia M. K. Spierings, who is a dermatologist and dermatological surgeon and the author of *Skintelligent: What You Really Need to Know to Get Great Skin* (Ebury Publishing, London, United Kingdom, 2022). She lives in London, United Kingdom, and Dubai, United Arab Emirates. Her website is DrNataliaSpierings.com.

He is married and lives with his wife, Maria, in the Greater Boston area of Massachusetts in the United States. He spends his free time playing samba and bossa nova guitar and horseback riding.

Index

B

D

E

F

G

I

J

K

L

M

N

O

P

Q

R

S

T

U

V

W

Z